TAKING CARE

Self-Care for 100 Common Symptoms and 20 Long-Term Ailments

by Michael B. Jacobs, M.D., and select faculty of the Stanford University School of Medicine

Medical Consultants
Primary Care: Michael B. Jacobs, MD, Professor of Medicine, Stanford University
Pediatrics: Jane A. Morton, MD, Clinical Professor of Pediatrics, Stanford University
Staff Physician, Palo Alto Medical Foundation, Palo Alto, California
OB-GYN: Maurice Druzin, MD, Professor of Gynecology and Obstetrics, Stanford University
Chief, Division of Maternal-Fetal Medicine, Stanford University
Geriatrics: Peter Pompei, MD, Associate Professor of Medicine, Stanford University
Director, Geriatric Medicine Fellowship Program, Stanford University

Managed Care Consultants
Robert Harmon, MD, MPH
Elizabeth Porter, MD, MPH
Bonnie Morcomb, RN, MS

Random House
New York

Taking Care is designed to help you make wise health care decisions and work more effectively with your health care provider. You should not rely on it, however, to replace necessary medical consultations to meet your individual health care needs.

Library of Congress Cataloging-in-Publication Data
Taking care: self-care for 100 common symptoms and 20 long-term ailments.
p.   cm.
ISBN 0-679-77794-6
1. Self-care, Health. 2. Medicine, Popular. I. Random House (Firm)
RA776.95.T35   1997
606—dc20   96-41153

Produced by CMD Publishing, a division of Current Medical Directions, Inc.
Illustrated by Patricia Shea

Random House website address: http://www.randomhouse.com/
Printed in the United States of America on acid-free paper
9876543

CONTENTS

Check this section for a quick
explanation of any of the words in
italics used throughout the book.

HOW TO USE THIS BOOK

This book was designed for people using managed care, as this seems to be the direction in which most health care is now heading. We have used the term "nurse information service" throughout the book for those people who have telephone access to a nurse as part of their health plan or through their employer. If you do not have a nurse information service, then simply call your doctor's office instead. We have used *italics* to flag words featured in the glossary on page 260.

The first section, "Take Charge of Your Health," provides key tips for getting the best out of your health care. It covers managed care plans, choosing a doctor, and keeping your medical costs down. In "Ten Strategies for a Healthy Lifestyle," you will learn essential information to help you and your family live a healthier life.

The 100 most common symptoms and problems are arranged alphabetically starting on page 29. They are listed by symptom (e.g., cough), by body area associated with a symptom (e.g., nose, runny), or by problem (e.g., splinter). You can also consult the index on page 265 for a full listing of the contents of the book.

Each entry contains all the information you will need at a glance, including a short description of the problem, an explanation of the most likely or important causes for the symptom, and a list of other causes (in order of prevalence) described elsewhere in the book.

The symptom chart for each entry is your most useful tool in deciding whether you need emergency assistance, a visit to the doctor, or whether you can manage the problem at home. If you work your way through the chart and do not find your particular circumstances described, call your nurse information service or doctor.

Self-care measures are outlined step-by-step to help you safely manage symptoms at home as appropriate. If over-the-counter medication is recommended, information on safe usage for pregnant women, children, and other special populations is provided. You will find this information located either in the section itself or, in the case of more widely used drugs, on page 27 in "Over-the-Counter Drug Information."

The "Prevention" section of each symptom gives you helpful pointers on how you can avoid this problem in the future. For many symptoms, you will find a special "Treating Your Child" section that includes vital information for the child in your care.

You will also find in-depth discussions of the 20 most common long-term ailments, arranged alphabetically starting on page 219. Each entry describes the disease and its management, with the emphasis on your role in the treatment plan and information on when you should seek medical help.

TAKE CHARGE OF YOUR HEALTH

The person most responsible for your state of health is you. As a knowledgeable, informed consumer of medical services, you can do a lot to prevent illness from striking, to prepare for problems should they occur, and to get the best treatment at the lowest cost.

Taking an active role in your health care requires a little effort—and some common sense. But the rewards are well worth it: less suffering from illness or injury; fewer visits to the doctor; less money spent on treatments, co-payments, and deductibles; greater productivity, vitality, and enjoyment of life.

Health and Safety at Home

Good health begins at home. Being prepared can prevent an emergency, so keep a well-stocked medicine cabinet and emergency supplies on hand. Here are some basic steps to take.

- Write down emergency phone numbers—doctor, ambulance, police, fire—and post them in a prominent place. Show all visitors and caretakers (e.g., grandparents or baby-sitters) where the list is. Teach your young children to dial 911 in case of an emergency.

- Check for and eliminate common household hazards, such as:
  - Faulty wiring or overloaded circuits
  - Cluttered storage areas (e.g., garage, attic, basement, hallways, or closets)
  - Paints, oil products, rags
  - Clogged chimneys or exhaust pipes
  - Loose flooring or rugs, especially on stairs
  - Top-heavy or wobbly furniture
  - Clutter on stairs

Your First-Aid Kit

Store the first-aid kit in a locked cabinet, away from children. It is also a good idea to stow a first-aid kit in each of the family cars. Kits should contain:

- Antacid
- Antibiotic cream or ointment (e.g., bacitracin)
- Antidiarrhea medication
- Antiseptic cream, lotion, or spray
- Calamine lotion (for rashes or itching)
- Eye patch
- Eye wash
- Flashlight
- Ipecac (to induce vomiting)
- Large gauze pads (to apply pressure to a large bleeding wound)
- Latex gloves
- Laxative
- Moistened sterile towelettes
- Needle
- Pain/fever medication such as aspirin or acetaminophen (*see* page 27)
- Petroleum jelly or other lubricant
- Rubbing alcohol or hydrogen peroxide
- Safety pins
- Safety razor blade
- Scissors
- Soap
- Square cloth of sufficient size to use as a sling
- Sterile adhesive bandages, gauze pads (4"x 4", 2"x 2"), adhesive tape
- Thermal blanket
- Thermometer
- Tongue depressors
- Tweezers

Your Rights

Being aware of your rights as a consumer of health care services will help you make smarter decisions when it comes to choosing a doctor, undergoing tests or procedures, or even negotiating terms of payment and insurance coverage. Exercising these rights can improve both the quality of your care and your satisfaction with it.

As a patient, you have the right:

- To be treated with dignity and respect at all times.
- To be told about your condition in clear and simple language.
- To have access to your medical records.
- To ask questions of your caregivers and to receive answers that you understand.
- To get second opinions.
- To be fully informed about the purpose, risks, and benefits of any test, procedure, or treatment.
- To refuse to undergo a test or treatment, even when it is recommended by your physician, after you have been fully informed.
- To know what alternative treatments are available and to know their risks and benefits.
- To know the costs of your treatment.
- To prepare a living will in which you define the type of medical treatment you do and do not accept.
- To designate a health care "proxy" or representative (e.g., a spouse, adult child, or close friend) who has the authority to make treatment decisions on your behalf should you be unable to do so yourself.
- To have confidentiality with respect to your medical records.
- To have privacy during examinations and conversations with health care providers.

- Keep the following in a locked cabinet and out of reach of children, or dispose of properly if no longer needed:
  - Poisons
  - Solvents
  - Cleaning agents
- Equip the house with smoke detectors and fire extinguishers on every floor. Test these devices every month to make sure that they are working. Replace batteries twice a year. Consider a carbon monoxide detector as well.
- If you have guns, lock them up unloaded.

Building a Relationship with Your Health Care Providers

Keep yourself healthy and practice self-care. Simple, common-sense treatments administered at home will often solve medical problems. Avoid the temptation to run to the doctor at the first sign of a sniffle or scratchy throat. By visiting physicians for appropriate reasons, you will show respect for their time and ability; in turn, you will receive careful attention for your real concerns. Choose your doctor carefully. If your insurance plan allows you a choice of physicians, take time to find a doctor with

The Best Doctor Is One Who:
- Is willing to listen to you
- Shows respect for you and your needs
- Treats the "whole you" rather than just your symptoms
- Explains the problem and its solution
- Earns your trust
- Respects your desire to get a second opinion
- Is available by phone to answer questions

whom you feel comfortable. Feeling mistrustful, anxious, or angry about your doctor is no way to build a relationship. Of course, your doctor should have adequate training and experience, but "bedside manner" counts for a lot.

Learn How to Communicate with Your Doctor.
To make the best use of your time during an office visit:

- Be on time. If it's your first visit, allow extra time to find the office and arrive early to complete any necessary registration material.
- Be ready to explain your problem clearly: what symptoms you are having, how and when the trouble began, and the treatment steps you have taken yourself, including alternative treatments.
- Write notes ahead of time. Avoid long-winded explanations and irrelevant details.
- Bring with you any important records: medical history, family details, previous treatments, and medication lists. Many physicians like to have these for review before the scheduled visit in order to maximize the time available for you at the visit.
- Prepare your list of questions in advance; keep the list short and to the point. An excessively long list can be distracting and defeating for the doctor and can waste valuable time.
- Be direct and honest. Discuss your main concern as well as anything that might be relevant to the problem, including use of other medications, your fears and concerns, and stressful events at home.
- Listen to what the doctor says. If it helps you, write notes or even tape-record the conversation.
- If you do not understand something, ask that it be repeated and explained. Sometimes you can speak to a nurse or other person in the office to get more complete (and less technical) answers.
- Ask for—and read—brochures or other written materials.

Understand the Treatment Plan.
If you receive a prescription, ask your doctor what the drug does, how to take it, and what side effects might arise. You can also ask your pharmacist—another important person on your health care team—some of these questions. If other treatments are prescribed, be clear about who is to perform them, when, and where. Make sure you know which follow-up steps to take, when to call and why, and with whom you should speak. Keep track of follow-up appointments, phone numbers, and other information. Many offices have a reminder system for follow-up appointments, but you should not depend on this. Assume this responsibility yourself.

Finding a Doctor

To locate names, ask:

- Your health plan administrator
- A referral service at a local hospital, county medical society, or academic medical center, etc.
- Family, friends, coworkers
- A nurse

To determine the nature of the practice, ask:

- If you can have a preliminary meeting to get acquainted
- What kind of patient load the physician has
- How difficult it is to schedule a "sick visit"
- How far in advance routine checkups or other "well visits" must be scheduled
- If the office has extended hours or 24-hour on-call coverage
- What kind of phone advice is available and with whom
- What services and other personnel are available
- How payment must be handled, whether a co-payment is required, if payments can be made in installments, etc.

To determine the doctor's style, look for:

- Good communication skills that suit your own style
- An ability to listen
- Signs that the physician is available to you and cares about your situation
- Patience and clarity when discussing treatments, alternative choices, risks, and benefits
- Willingness to let you ask questions and to supply clear, thorough answers
- A philosophy of prevention and education
- Friendly, helpful office personnel
- Adequate staff support
- An office that is clean, pleasant, well organized, and comfortable

Medical Services and Settings.

Getting care from the right place at the right time is crucial both for good health and for keeping costs down. You should not visit the emergency room to have a splinter removed, nor should you check into a hospital for routine X rays. Emergency rooms are designed to handle emergencies and not routine care. Using an emergency room for routine care is costly and the waiting period can be considerable.

Make sure you understand what types of care your insurance plan covers. For example, your insurer may not cover emergency-room treatment for minor problems and may not reimburse you for visits to specialists that have not been authorized in advance.

Share in Medical Decision-Making.

Ask why a treatment or test is recommended. Tell the doctor what kind of treatment you prefer. If a medication causes intolerable side effects, or if treatment is interfering with your quality of life, let the physician know. Discuss whether alternative therapies are available. Remember, though, that by sharing in this process you accept your share of responsibility for following the treatment plan and for staying in touch with your doctor about the outcome.

Medical Care Settings

Ambulance: A vehicle for transporting a seriously ill or injured person. Ambulance personnel are trained to administer first aid or emergency treatment either in the home or en route to the hospital to people who are unconscious or bleeding, who are experiencing difficulty breathing, who have symptoms of heart attack or seizures lasting several minutes, or who may have neck or spinal injuries.

Diagnostic clinic or suite: A facility offering X rays, radiological tests, ultrasound, or other tests and procedures not provided by a physician and not requiring hospitalization.

Doctor's office: A suite of rooms where physicians or other staff conduct physical examinations, patient interviews, diagnostic tests, and procedures that do not require hospitalization or general anesthesia.

Emergency room: Hospital facility designed for handling crises that pose an immediate threat to life or limb, such as major injury, severe bleeding, heart attacks or strokes, severe pain, difficulty breathing, or mental confusion. The ER is not a place for treating bumps, bruises, or sore throats; for providing continuing care of chronic illnesses; or for performing complex diagnostic tests.

Home health care: Treatment administered in the patient's home. In many cases, people with chronic conditions can be treated at home more conveniently, more pleasantly, and less expensively. Home health care usually requires special equipment, part-time or live-in nurses, or family members or volunteers who have been trained to help.

Hospice care: Treatment offered to terminally ill patients and delivered at a special facility or in the patient's home. Hospices provide medical treatment, but their main purpose is to ease pain and suffering and to provide an environment that is more comfortable than the hospital's.

Hospital: A medical facility providing around-the-clock medical and surgical treatment for severe illness; supervised recovery from serious injury; and presurgical treatment, surgery, and postoperative recovery.

Long-term care facility: A nursing home or rehabilitation (convalescent) center offering care for the elderly or for people recovering from illness or injury who do not need hospitalization but who need help caring for themselves or performing basic tasks of daily living.

Surgery center: A facility (separate from the hospital) that offers surgical treatment for uncomplicated problems that do not require lengthy stays, either for presurgical preparation or postoperative recovery.

Urgent care (walk-in or drop-in) clinic: Neighborhood facility offering quick treatment for simple illnesses or injuries. Clinics are open long hours and no appointment is usually needed. This is a great alternative for an emergency room when the situation is not life-threatening.

Know Your Health Plan

There are many different types of insurance plans. Understanding the options available will make you a better consumer and help you get the most out of your health care coverage.

The traditional form of insurance is known as a fee-for-service or indemnity plan. In this pay-as-you-go system, the provider issues you a bill for each visit or procedure. Usually you pay the fee directly, then submit a claim to the insurer, who pays you back for covered expenses. More comprehensive plans also cover expenses for prescription medications, psychiatric treatment, and dental care.

Today most insurance plans fall under the broad category of managed care, which is designed to hold down the rising costs of health care. The various plans are organized somewhat differently. Generally, the concept is that the company enters into an agreement with one or more physicians or hospitals (also called providers) to hold the line on costs. In some plans, the contract stipulates that providers will be paid a certain amount each month for each patient who signs onto the plan. These are called capitated plans, because they pay providers "per capita," or "per head." In other plans, known as discounted fee-for-service plans, providers agree to charge a lower rate in exchange for being sent a higher volume of patients. Insurers also negotiate with drug companies to supply medications and hospital supplies at volume discounts. These savings are then passed along to patients in the form of lower premiums.

The main incentives for patients to enroll in a managed care plan are lower premium expenses, unlimited doctor visits, and freedom from insurance claim problems. For some people, the major concern about managed care is whether the plan allows them to see the doctors they prefer. Insurers try to address that concern by recruiting as many qualified health care providers as possible. Certain types of plans (but not all of them) reimburse members regardless of which doctor they see, although payment may be at a higher rate if a patient receives care from a participating provider. Another issue involving managed care is whether such policies restrict the treatment options available. In general, managed care plans are designed to help physicians and patients choose treatments that are proven to create the best results and that are delivered in the most appropriate setting at the most reasonable cost.

Seven Ways to Control Medical Costs

Live a Healthy Life.

The best strategy for avoiding medical bills is prevention. Even the simple act of washing your hands after using the toilet or before preparing food can significantly reduce the spread of disease. Be sure that you, your children, and elderly relatives receive recommended vaccinations at the right times. *See* "Ten Strategies for a Healthy Lifestyle," page 16.

Care for Yourself.

In many cases, a minor illness can be managed successfully at home until it runs its course. Keep this book handy and use it before making an appointment with your doctor. Call the doctor's office or nurse information service for guidance; on their advice, try over-the-counter remedies; rest;

wait a day or so to see if the problem gets better. If your illness is contagious, avoid exposing others to germs.

Understand Your Health Care Plan.

Know what is covered and what is not. Be sure that you know whether your plan requires preauthorization for hospital stays or diagnostic tests. Keep track of insurance bills and payments to make sure that you are reimbursed appropriately.

Prepare for Doctor's Visits.

Keep your own medical diary to write down doctor visits, medical tests, names of medications, and prescription numbers. This saves time during appointments and avoids confusion or duplication of services. Before the appointment, be ready to describe your complaint clearly, make sure any relevant medical records are available, and write down your questions beforehand.

Use Medical Resources Appropriately.

Emergency-room services are for true emergencies, not for routine care or for treatment of minor complaints. Start your treatment process by seeing primary care physicians first. They can handle most medical problems, and they will refer you to a specialist when necessary. Before undergoing any medical test or procedure, ask why it is being done and whether it is necessary. Avoid costly hospitalizations. Today, thanks to advances in technology, many procedures that once required hospitalization can be done more quickly, safely, and cheaply in the doctor's office.

Reduce Drug Costs.

Before filling a prescription, understand what the drug is for and how it is used. Don't insist on drugs when your physician recommends otherwise (e.g., antibiotics for a cold or viral illness). Ask about side effects, especially those that may be so serious that you quit taking the medication. (Buying a drug that you do not or cannot take is a waste of money.) Tell your doctor about any other drugs you are using (including alcohol or illegal drugs) to avoid interactions. Ask whether a generic version of the drug is available, since such products are usually cheaper than their brand-name counterparts. Shop around for the lowest price on a drug. Follow directions exactly. Never stop taking a drug without talking to your doctor first.

Watch Out for Quacks.

People who get sick will often do anything or try anything to get better. There are many unscrupulous individuals and companies out there who prey on the fears of the desperately ill by promoting phony, worthless, or downright dangerous treatments. Resist the temptation to buy products that feature personal testimonials from patients or celebrities, that claim to contain "miraculous" or "secret" ingredients, that have not been evaluated in scientific tests, that promise to cure dozens of diseases, and that are available only by mail. Also be wary of physicians who prescribe the same treatment for every patient, regardless of the diagnosis, who promise treatments with "no risk," or who suggest doing things that are unethical or illegal.

Health Care Plans:
A Quick Guide to Types and Terms

Co-payment: A small fee (usually $5 or $10) you must pay every time you visit the doctor or buy a prescription medication. Managed care plans allow providers to collect co-payments as a way of reducing unnecessary visits for minor or routine illnesses.

EPO (Exclusive Provider Organization): A managed care plan that reimburses you only if you obtain health care from certain providers.

Fee-for-Service (or Indemnity) Plan: Standard insurance coverage in which you usually pay the provider for care, file a claim, and are reimbursed by the carrier. Usually these plans pay you a percentage of costs (typically 80%) until you meet the annual deductible; after that point you are reimbursed in full until you reach the limits of coverage for that particular type of care.

HMO (Health Maintenance Organization): A prepaid insurance plan, often one that hires or contracts with its own physicians to provide medical care to members. Some HMOs are capitated (i.e., they pay doctors a fixed rate per member), but others combine various elements of managed care, such as discounted fees for service. If you participate in an HMO, you generally receive care only from the physicians who work for that HMO, except in emergencies.

MSA (Medical Savings Account): A plan in which one part of your premium pays for an insurance policy covering you for catastrophic illness and the other part is put into a fund to cover routine care. You may spend this money as you wish for medical treatment; anything left over at the end of the year is yours to keep.

Out-of-Pocket Service: Treatment for which you pay the provider directly, without being reimbursed by an insurer.

POS (Point of Service) Plan: Insurance that lets you choose the type of reimbursement you prefer at the time you go for treatment. For example, if you are dealing with routine illness, you may elect to see any provider who offers a discounted fee, but if you have a serious illness, you may elect to see a specialist of your own choosing. In that case, you will still be reimbursed, but at a lower rate. POS plans offer the advantage of flexibility but at an overall higher cost.

PPO (Preferred Provider Organization): A plan in which members receive a list of doctors and hospitals (the "preferred providers") who have agreed to provide their services at a significant discount. If you get treatment from these providers, you will be charged less (or will be reimbursed at a higher rate) than if you get treatment from a nonparticipant.

TEN STRATEGIES FOR A HEALTHY LIFESTYLE

1. Drink Alcohol in Moderation

Alcohol is an important element in rituals and traditions, and it may offer certain health benefits in some people. But alcohol is also a powerful drug and, like any drug, it can be abused. If you choose to drink alcohol, the key to maintaining a healthy lifestyle is moderation.

Know the Alcohol Content of Different Beverages.
A 12-ounce beer contains as much alcohol as a 4-ounce glass of wine or 1 ounce of distilled liquor.

Do Not Mix Alcohol and Drugs.
Many prescription and over-the-counter medications can interact with alcohol and cause serious problems and sometimes death. Ask your pharmacist if your prescription is affected by alcohol. Combining illegal drugs and alcohol is especially dangerous.

Do Not Drink and Drive.
Alcohol impairs judgment, muscle control, and vision. If you have been drinking, ask another person to drive or arrange for other transportation. Never ride as a passenger with a driver who has been drinking.

If You Are Pregnant, Do Not Drink at All.
Alcohol can damage the fetus.

Do Not Expect Coffee or a Cold Shower to Sober You Up.
The effects of drinking only wear off after the body has had enough time to metabolize the alcohol and remove it from the bloodstream.

Do Not Feel Pressured to Drink.
Well-meaning hosts may encourage you to drink more than you want or need. If polite refusals are not enough, simply keep your glass filled with water or soda and sip it slowly. If you do not feel comfortable around people who are drinking heavily, leave.

Do Not Make Drinking a Habit.
One to 2 drinks a day may not pose a major health risk, but routine drinking (e.g., every day at the same time) is a warning signal of a possible overdependence on alcohol. This is treatable. Ask your nurse information service or doctor about getting help.

2. Check Up on Your Health

Catching health problems before they become serious is an important strategy for staying well and living long.

Know the Factors That Affect the Impact of Alcohol.

- Food in your stomach slows down the rate at which alcohol enters the bloodstream. Eat before drinking, and eat something while drinking.
- Pace yourself. One drink per hour with a 2-drink maximum is a good policy.
- People with smaller bodies are more vulnerable to alcohol. A 100-pound person may feel more intoxicated after 1 drink than a 200-pound person does after 2.
- Women are generally more susceptible to alcohol than men, regardless of weight.

Get Regular Medical Checkups.

A physical examination at regular intervals, depending on your age, medical history, and doctor's recommendation, is important. During the exam you may need several simple screening tests or procedures, depending on your general health, age, and personal risk factors, such as a family history of a disease. You may undergo procedures such as height and weight measurements, blood pressure readings, blood tests to measure cholesterol, and stool tests for blood. Women patients undergo a cervical (Pap) smear, careful breast exam, and mammograms to detect *cancer*. You can help your doctor by reporting any unusual lumps or changes in the skin, breast, or testicles. Your doctor should inquire and counsel you about certain health risks, such as problem drinking, tobacco use, diet, exercise, safe sex, substance abuse, dental health, eye health, and injury prevention.

Ask Your Doctor about Immunizations.

All infants and children should be immunized against various diseases, including *diphtheria*, *pertussis*, *tetanus*, polio, haemophilus *influenza* type B, *measles*, mumps (*see* page 196), rubella, chicken pox, and *hepatitis* B. Women planning pregnancies should review their immunization status before trying to conceive. If you are over 65 or suffering from a chronic disease, you may need immunizations against *influenza* and *pneumonia*. Travelers should get all necessary shots before leaving the country.

3. Eat Healthfully

A proper diet can help prevent illness and promote healing should illness strike. Here are some general tips on how to eat right:

Select Foods That Provide Important Nutrients.

By eating a variety of foods in the right proportions, you will provide your bones, tissues,

Eat a Variety of Foods

The five main food groups (and the suggested numbers of daily servings) are:

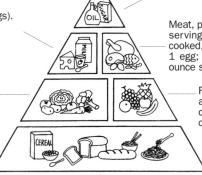

Fats, oils, and sweets should be used sparingly.

Milk, yogurt, and cheese (2–3 servings). One serving might be 1 cup of milk, 1 1/2 ounces of natural cheese, or 2 ounces of processed cheese.

Meat, poultry, fish, dry beans, eggs, and nuts (2–4 servings). One serving might be 2-3 ounces of cooked, lean meat; 1/2 cup of cooked dry beans; 1 egg; or 2 tablespoons of peanut butter. A 9-ounce steak contains 3 servings.

Vegetables (3–5 servings). One serving might be 1 cup of raw, leafy vegetables; 1/2 cup of other vegetables, cooked or raw; or 3/4 cup of vegetable juice.

Fruit (2–4 servings). One serving might be an apple, banana, or orange; 1/2 cup of chopped, cooked, or canned fruit; or 3/4 cup of fruit juice.

Bread, cereal, rice, and pasta (6–11 servings). One serving might be a slice of bread; 1 ounce of ready-to-eat cereal; or 1/2 cup of cooked cereal, rice, or pasta. A large plate of spaghetti contains several servings.

Adapted from the U.S. Department of Agriculture's Food Guide Pyramid.

and organs with the various substances they need to function.

In general, a good diet is made up of:

- Proteins—about 10–15% of calories.
- Carbohydrates—at least 50% of calories.
- Fats—less than 30% of calories. Saturated fat (i.e., fat from animal products) should provide less than 10% of calories, and cholesterol should be less than 300 mg.
- Fiber—a recommended daily intake is 25–30 grams daily, which can be found in dried apricots, whole-grain flour, celery, raisins, bran, and other fruits and vegetables.
- Vitamins and minerals—there are 13 major vitamins needed by the body (e.g., A, B6, C, and D) and 13 major minerals (e.g., calcium, sodium, and iron). Good sources include carrots; green, leafy vegetables; citrus fruits; whole-grain products; fish; and lean meats. Ask your nurse information service or doctor about how much of these nutrients your diet should contain.

Watch Calories.

Calories are measures of food's energy content. A standard daily diet provides 2,000–2,500 calories (varying with your weight and usual level of activity); more important than the number of calories is the need to maintain balance between energy consumed and energy burned. Excess (unused) calories become excess body weight.

Select Whole, Unprocessed Foods.

Brown rice, fresh vegetables, and whole-grain breads are better than white rice, canned vegetables, or breads made with bleached, processed flours.

Drink Liquids, Especially Water.

Try to drink about 6–8 glasses of water a day. Avoid coffee and alcohol.

Watch Fat and Cholesterol.

Use unsaturated fats (those that are liquid at room temperature) such as corn, safflower, or sunflower oils, rather than saturated fats (e.g., lard, butter, and shortening). Use cooking techniques such as steaming or microwaving, which do not require fats, rather than frying or sautéing. Limit your consumption of foods with cholesterol and fat. Choose skim or 1% milk and use nonfat or low-fat dairy products. Eat no more than 6 ounces per day of lean meat, fish, or skinless poultry, and eat no more than 3 or 4 eggs per week (including eggs in prepared foods such as store-bought cakes). Avoid shellfish (e.g., shrimp or lobster) and organ meats (e.g., liver or gizzards), which are high in cholesterol.

Reduce Sugar and Salt.

Sugar supplies calories and little else, nutritionally. Too much salt (sodium) may contribute to high blood pressure (*see* page 244), blood vessel disease (*see* page 51), and fluid retention.

Maintain Good Eating Habits.

Do not skip meals; eating smaller meals spread out through the day is healthier than eating one large meal. Eat healthy snacks. Do not become a slave to a diet; allow yourself treats; eat moderate amounts.

Be Cautious About Food Supplements.
A healthy, balanced diet usually provides all the nutrients needed. Vitamin and mineral supplements are seldom necessary. However, menstruating women may need extra iron and the elderly often need calcium supplements to guard against osteoporosis (*see* page 250). Check with your nurse information service or doctor before taking supplements. More is not necessarily better and can even be dangerous.

4. Prevent Drug Abuse

Any drug carries with it the risk of abuse. Illegal drugs such as marijuana, cocaine, and heroin are dangerous because they damage the body and the mind and because they can be highly addictive. Even legal drugs—including prescription medications and over-the-counter products—can be misused. A key strategy for staying healthy is to avoid using any illegal drugs and to use all medications only as directed.

Learn the Facts.
Education is the best way to prevent drug abuse. Ask your doctor or librarian for information and share what you learn with others in your family. Talk openly and honestly with your children about the problem. When people understand the risks involved, they are less likely to misuse drugs.

Avoid Situations That Can Promote Drug Abuse.
Do not attend parties or events where drugs are used. Avoid boredom; develop interests and goals; structure your time so that you have plenty of activities to keep you busy.

Know the Warning Signs of Substance Abuse.
In adolescents, signs include:

- Abandonment of former friends or activities in favor of a peer group that uses or approves of drugs
- Parents who abuse drugs
- An attitude that drug use is harmless and acceptable
- Rebellious behavior
- Truancy; poor or declining school performance
- Lying about whereabouts and activities
- Sudden strong mood changes
- Abusive behavior and angry outbursts
- Brushes with the law

- Drug paraphernalia in the bedroom or car
- Physical symptoms such as fatigue, lethargy, chronic cough, red eyes, frequent headaches

In adults, signs may include some of the above as well as:

- Chronic health problems
- Money troubles
- Problems at work: lateness, absences, poor performance, frequent job changes
- Violent or suicidal behavior
- Frequent accidents at work, at home, or in the car
- Trouble with the law
- Loss of interest in hobbies or socializing

Use Medications Only as Directed.
Follow instructions carefully. Take doses in the right amounts at the time indicated. If you skip a dose call your pharmacist or nurse information service for instructions. Avoid alcohol while using medication. Dispose of medicines whose expiration dates have passed by flushing them down the toilet. Never take medicines prescribed for someone else.

5. Exercise

Exercise is vital to a healthy lifestyle. It tones and strengthens muscles, increases stamina, strengthens the heart, improves circulation, lowers blood pressure, improves digestion, burns excess calories, facilitates sleep, promotes resistance to disease, and enhances your ability to recover from illness. In addition to its physical benefits, exercise improves mood, releases stress, and increases mental alertness. By improving your personal appearance, exercise can also boost confidence and self-esteem.

Check with Caregivers Before Beginning an Exercise Program.
You need to know if you have any medical conditions, such as a heart condition, that might affect your ability to exercise. Ask your care providers to suggest exercises best suited to your interests, needs, and general state of health.

Choose Exercises That You Enjoy.
If you like what you're doing, chances are you'll stick with it longer. If you cannot stand jogging, for example, swim or bike.

Begin Gradually.
Start with moderate goals, then increase the intensity and frequency of exercise by about 10% a week as your stamina improves. If you feel pain or stress, ease up.

Use the Right Equipment.
Wear athletic shoes designed for the type of exercise that you are doing. Avoid injury by asking for instructions on how to use weight machines, stationary bicycles, or other equipment.

Try to Exercise the Whole Body.
Design a varied, all-around program that exercises both the upper and the lower body. Aerobic exercise such as running, dancing, or bicycling builds stamina by increasing the work load on the heart and the lungs; weight training strengthens specific muscles; calisthenics can strengthen joints and keep them limber.

Warm Up and Cool Down.
Muscles need to be stretched and conditioned before undergoing vigorous activity. Take time (at least 5 minutes) to limber up; after exercise, allow time to cool off.

Make Exercise Part of Your Routine.
A good goal is to perform vigorous exercise for 20–30 minutes, 3 or 4 times a week. If you plan your exercise on the same days at the same time, it will be easier for you to stick to the schedule. If this is not possible, make the most of your daily routine by walking briskly around the home or office and performing daily tasks with extra vigor.

Find an "Exercise Buddy."
Many people find it much easier to stay with an exercise program if they invite a friend to join them.

Allow Intervals of Rest Between Exercise Days.
Taking a few days off each week prevents musculoskeletal injury and helps sustain commitment to an exercise program.

6. Stay Safe

Avoiding injuries, accidents, and illness is often a matter of common sense. Following are some suggestions for reducing risks in the home and outdoors.

Wear Protective Equipment During Sporting Activities.
Skaters need helmets and elbow and knee guards; baseball and softball players should wear batting helmets; bicyclists and motorcyclists should wear protective headgear. Eye protection is recommended for racquet sports.

Avoid Overexposure to Sunlight.
To reduce skin *cancer* risk, use sunblock with a sun protection formula (SPF) of 15 or higher. Wear hats and sunglasses to protect your eyes.

Prevent Falls or Accidents in the Home.

- Keep hallways and staircases clear of clutter and secure rugs and carpets to avoid trips and falls.
- Use nightlights in bathrooms and hallways.
- Make sure paints, solvents, and oil products are stored in appropriate, sealed containers away from rags or papers.
- Use stepladders, not chairs or stools, to reach high places.

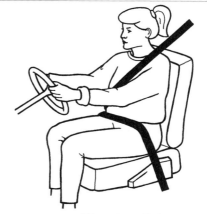

Wear Seat Belts.
Everyone in the car—driver and passengers, front seat and back—should always wear seat belts, even in cars with air bags. Always use lap belts. Do not carry more passengers than there are seat belts. Infants and children need special car seats, which should always be installed in the back seat.

Practice Household Fire-Prevention Measures.
- Have household wiring inspected.
- Discard or repair any electric cords, plugs, or outlets that are worn or uncovered.
- Never touch uncovered wires.
- Do not overload circuits by using multiple outlet adaptors or extension cords.
- Use only polarized plugs.
- Install smoke detectors (and possibly carbon monoxide detectors) in different locations. Test them periodically and replace batteries when needed.
- Have a fire extinguisher.
- Have an escape plan.

> **If You Have Children in the House:**
> - Keep corrosive chemicals, charcoal fire starters, and other flammables locked away in a safe place.
> - Cook on the back burners of the stove and turn all pot handles in.
> - Keep dangerous objects (e.g., knives, cleaning products, or medications) out of children's reach.
> - Teach your children about fire safety and handling fire hazards.
> - Put safety caps on outlets and extension cords.

Practice Safe Sex.

Unless you are in a monogamous (i.e., mutually faithful) relationship and have tested free of infection for sexually transmitted diseases (STDs), you will need to use latex condoms, preferably ones that are treated with the spermicide nonoxynol-9 and that have a reservoir on the end, each and every time you have sex. Although condoms are effective against STDs, they do not provide 100% protection. Sexual practices such as anal intercourse or oral sex also pose a high risk for transmitting STDs. The risk of acquiring and transmitting HIV infection is higher among certain groups: those who have had homosexual sex, blood disorders, or blood transfusions; prostitutes; injection drug users who share needles; and those who have had sex with numerous partners or anyone in a high-risk group.

Know Emergency Procedures and Phone Numbers.
Plan fire escape routes and conduct emergency drills. Keep emergency phone numbers (e.g., police, fire, and medical) beside every phone. Make sure all family members, even children, know how to call for help.

7. Get Good Sleep

Sleep keeps the body strong and the mind alert. Many people are chronically sleep deprived, and they consequently suffer from physical ailments, mental problems, injuries, and accidents. Follow these steps to get the rest you need.

Exercise and Eat Right.

Getting appropriate exercise (but not in the 3 hours before bedtime) helps promote sleep. So does eating a healthy diet, maintaining a healthy weight, and following a regular meal schedule. Some foods, such as turkey and dairy products, contain tryptophan, which may promote sleep.

Limit Caffeine Intake.

Coffee, tea, colas, chocolate, many cold and pain relievers, and diet aids contain caffeine which keeps you awake. Switch to decaffeinated beverages. Avoid caffeine in the evening.

Stop Smoking (*see* page 24).

Nicotine is a stimulant; cravings for cigarettes can also cause you to stay awake.

Reduce Your Consumption of Alcohol (*see* page 16).
Many people drink a "nightcap" to help them sleep. However, when the effects of alcohol wear off a few hours later, there is a risk that you will wake up again.

Maintain a Healthy Sleep Environment.
Replace uncomfortable mattresses and pillows. Make sure the bedroom is as quiet and dark as possible. Use a noise filter to shut out sounds from the outside. Keep the temperature cool, and use a humidifier if necessary. Wear loose, comfortable, lightweight sleepwear.

Practice a Good Sleep Routine.
Lie down to sleep at the same time every night and rise at the same time in the morning. Avoid naps during the daytime. Do not eat heavy meals or undergo strenuous exercise shortly before bedtime. Warm baths (not brisk showers) can be soothing.

Put Your Mind to Rest.
Anxiety and depression (*see* page 238) can interfere with sleep.

Use Sleep Medications Cautiously, if at All.
There are many prescription and over-the-counter (OTC) products available to help you fall asleep. If you must take these drugs, do so cautiously. Use only appropriate doses and do not mix drugs and alcohol. Use OTC sleep medications no more than twice a week and for no longer than 2 weeks. If you need them for longer periods, talk to a doctor or call your nurse information service.

8. Manage Your Stress and Anxiety

Stress is the body's physical response to excessive demands, frequent changes in routine, or a threat to life or limb. Anxiety is an emotional response to stress. Unrelieved stress can lead to a range of health complaints: weakened immunity, heart conditions, digestive disorders, muscle fatigue and tension, skin problems, breathing difficulties, and so on. The better you cope with stress and anxiety—or better yet, prevent stress from becoming too severe in the first place—the healthier you will be. Here are some general guidelines.

Identify the Problem.
Figure out what is causing stress and anxiety: a life change (e.g., moving, a new job, a new baby, or aging); a loss (e.g., divorce, a death in the family, or getting fired); a physical ailment (e.g., *cancer* or a severe infection); or excessive demands and overwork. If there is a medical problem, seek appropriate treatment. If it is a psychological issue, you may need help from a therapist, counselor, or support group.

Practice Relaxation Techniques.
When you are under stress, your muscles tighten, causing neck, back, or chest pain and making breathing harder. Paying attention to breathing helps muscles relax. Lie or sit comfortably, close your eyes and breathe in slowly, hold your breath for a few seconds, and exhale slowly. Continue for 5 minutes or more. Long walks, warm baths, meditating, or just sitting quietly can also be soothing.

Use Medications with Caution.

Antianxiety drugs can relieve anxiety quickly and effectively, tranquilizers can calm you down, and antidepressants can help you cope with low moods. However, these medications have side effects and can be abused. Use these products carefully, following your physician's advice. Remember that drugs may relieve your symptoms, but the underlying cause of stress and anxiety still needs to be addressed.

Work on Changing Attitudes and Behavior.

Do not dwell on negative thoughts or past events. Think positively and look to the future. Focus on one issue at a time, create a plan to address the problem, and take action. Break down tasks and problems into individual, easily accomplished steps, so that things do not seem so overwhelming. Stay active socially, since being with close friends can relieve stress. Talk about your concerns with a trusted friend or relative. Stress sometimes arises from frequent changes in routine; establishing and following daily patterns can help. Do not go to bed angry; try to resolve conflicts first.

9. Avoid Tobacco

Use of tobacco is this country's leading cause of preventable illness and premature death. Do not start using tobacco in any form, or if you already use it, quit.

Do Not Start.

When people start smoking, they experience coughing, headaches, and dizziness. If you pay attention to your body's warnings, you won't get hooked!

Teach Your Children.

Youngsters face a lot of pressure to start smoking. Their peers may believe smoking is "cool" or grown-up. Media advertising and celebrities make smoking seem glamorous. Adolescents are highly vulnerable to such pressures. Parents should set an example by not smoking and should talk frankly with youngsters about tobacco.

Make the Decision to Quit.

The first requirement is motivation. Be firmly committed to giving up the habit completely. Cutting down on the number of cigarettes should not be your ultimate goal.

Know the Dangers.

People who are informed about the health risks of tobacco are less likely to start using it or are more motivated to quit.

- Tobacco causes *cancer*, emphysema (*see* page 232), bronchitis (*see* page 232), and heart disease (*see* page 236).
- Snuff, chewing tobacco, and "smokeless tobacco" cause cancer of the mouth and tongue. These forms of tobacco are no less dangerous than smoking.
- Secondhand or passive smoke endangers nonsmokers.
- Nicotine, the main drug in tobacco, is highly addictive, physically and psychologically.

Make a Plan to Quit Smoking.

- Set a deadline and stick to it.
- Make a list of your reasons for quitting.
- If necessary, use nicotine gum or skin patches, which deliver a regulated and gradually diminishing dose of the drug, to avoid withdrawal symptoms.
- Consider hypnotism, acupuncture, or participation in support groups.
- Recruit friends and family to support your effort.
- Exercise.
- Snack on vegetables, suck on candies, or chew gum as a smoking substitute.
- Anticipate weight gain. Most people who quit do put on a few pounds, partly because their *metabolism* slows down and partly because they eat more as a way to satisfy addictive cravings. A few extra pounds are much less of a health risk than smoking.
- Reward yourself for success: Use the money you would have spent on cigarettes to buy yourself a present.

Go Smoke-Free.

You will send a strong message if you declare your home smoke-free. Most smokers will understand and comply.

10. Control Your Weight

Excess body weight endangers health in a number of ways. It strains the heart and taxes the circulation, adds stress to bones and muscles, complicates breathing, and increases the risk of other diseases such as diabetes (*see* page 240), *cancer*, and high blood pressure (*see* page 244). The figures on page 26 show the acceptable range of weight for men and women of different heights.

Strike a Balance.

The key to weight management is achieving a balance between the calories you consume and the calories you burn off during the day. If you want to lose weight, eat less and increase your level of physical activity. (Being too thin poses its own health risks: loss of menstrual periods in women, digestive problems, hormonal imbalances, loss of sex drive and fertility, and irregular heartbeats.)

Eat Less.

A typical American consumes more calories than needed. A standard diet is 2,000–2,500 calories a day. As a guideline, eating 500–1,000 fewer calories than you expend per day typically results in a weight loss of about a pound per week.

Eat Sensibly.

Avoid second helpings; skip desserts (or eat fruit); eat smaller meals on a regular schedule rather than eating one large meal a day or skipping meals; cut down on snacks; eat only when hungry. Do not read or watch television while eating; eat slowly (put your fork down between bites); be aware of "hidden" calories (e.g., alcohol); use smaller plates (it makes the portions look larger).

Avoid Fats.

Ounce for ounce, fat contains the highest concentrations of calories. Reduce the amount of red meat, nuts, pastries, sauces, salad dressings, butter, and oils in your diet. Replace them with whole-grain foods, poultry, pasta, and so on. Do not use fats in cooking; bake, broil, or microwave food instead.

Exercise.

Vigorous exercise provides many benefits. It burns off calories and helps replace fatty tissue with muscular tissue. Aerobic exercise may speed up *metabolism*, making your body more efficient at using energy. Walk, climb stairs, garden—any activity helps use up calories.

Be Patient.

Weight loss requires time. You may lose weight relatively quickly in the first few weeks because of fluid loss, but the rate of loss will slow down afterwards. Once you get to your desired weight, maintain it through careful diet and exercise.

Avoid Fad or "Crash" Diets.

Starvation diets, very-low-calorie liquid diets (under 1,000 calories per day), and other such strategies can be dangerous. Talk to your health care professionals about developing a sensible weight loss strategy.

Male weight/height

128 lb	5'1"	150 lb
130 lb	5'2"	153 lb
132 lb	5'3"	156 lb
134 lb	5'4"	160 lb
136 lb	5'5"	164 lb
138 lb	5'6"	168 lb
140 lb	5'7"	172 lb
142 lb	5'8"	176 lb
144 lb	5'9"	180 lb
146 lb	5'10"	184 lb
149 lb	5'11"	188 lb
152 lb	6'0"	192 lb
155 lb	6'1"	197 lb
158 lb	6'2"	202 lb
162 lb	6'3"	207 lb

Female weight/height

102 lb	4'9"	131 lb
103 lb	4'10"	134 lb
104 lb	4'11"	137 lb
106 lb	5'	140 lb
108 lb	5'1"	143 lb
111 lb	5'2"	147 lb
114 lb	5'3"	151 lb
117 lb	5'4"	155 lb
120 lb	5'5"	159 lb
123 lb	5'6"	163 lb
126 lb	5'7"	167 lb
129 lb	5'8"	170 lb
132 lb	5'9"	173 lb
135 lb	5'10"	176 lb
138 lb	5'11"	179 lb

Adapted from the MetLife Height and Weight Table, Statistical Bulletin, 1983. Copyright © 1983, 1993, Metropolitan Life Insurance Co.

OVER-THE-COUNTER DRUG INFORMATION

Important Information About OTC Medication:

- Do not buy drugs if the packaging or seal has been tampered with.
- Check that products in your medicine cabinet have not passed their expiration date.
- Follow the directions written on the package and do not exceed the recommended dose. Call your pharmacist or the manufacturer's toll-free number if you have any questions.
- Cold and flu preparations often contain combinations of over-the-counter medications.
- Check the active ingredients listed on the package label and look for warnings that apply to your medical history. Remember that your pharmacist is available for all your questions about prescription and/or over-the-counter medications.
- Never take medication in the dark.
- Do not mix medications or transfer them from their original containers.
- Store medications in a cool, dry place to avoid moisture unless otherwise directed by a health care professional.
- Do not combine over-the-counter medications with prescription or other medications without discussing it first with a health care professional.

Acetaminophen

- Taking the manufacturer's recommended doses of acetaminophen is considered relatively safe if you are pregnant or breast-feeding. However, check with your nurse information service or doctor before using this product.
- Do not use acetaminophen if you have kidney or liver disease, viral infections of the liver, or if you regularly fast or drink alcohol.
- Do not take acetaminophen for more than 10 consecutive days if you have no fever (5 days for children) or 3 days if you have a fever, unless prescribed by your doctor.
- If you cannot digest phenylalanine, be aware that some chewable acetaminophen contains aspartame which breaks down into phenylalanine during *metabolism*.
- If you smoke, you may need a higher dose of acetaminophen; call your nurse information service or doctor, or ask your pharmacist.

Aspirin

- If you are pregnant, or may become pregnant, you should consult your doctor before using aspirin. It is especially important not to use aspirin during the last 3 months of pregnancy unless specifically directed to do so by a doctor because it may cause problems in the fetus or complications during delivery.
- Do not give aspirin to anyone under 19 years of age! It may cause a rare but serious problem called Reye's syndrome. Instead, use ibuprofen or acetaminophen for fever or pain as your health professional recommends.
- Do not use aspirin if you have liver damage, a history of peptic *ulcers*, or any bleeding disorder. If you have asthma or are scheduled for surgery, check with your doctor before using aspirin.
- Do not use aspirin if you are taking a prescription drug for anticoagulation (thinning the blood), diabetes, gout, or arthritis, or if you are taking

zidovudine (AZT) for AIDS, unless directed by a doctor.

- Do not take aspirin for more than 10 consecutive days if you have no fever or 3 days if you have a fever, unless prescribed by your doctor.
- Take aspirin with food, milk, or water (or look for "enteric coated" on the package) to reduce stomach irritation.

Hydrocortisone Cream

- If you are pregnant, or may become pregnant, you should consult your doctor before using hydrocortisone cream.
- Consult your doctor before using hydrocortisone cream on infants and children. If used on large areas or over long periods of time, it increases the risk of absorption into the bloodstream and possible adverse side effects.
- Do not use hydrocortisone cream if you have severe kidney disease, diabetes, *tuberculosis*, or a history of peptic *ulcers*.
- Do not use hydrocortisone cream if you are using a topical antibacterial or antifungal drug without first checking with your nurse information service, doctor, or pharmacist.
- Avoid contact with the eyes.

Nonsteroidal Anti-inflammatory Drugs (NSAIDs)

- Ibuprofen, ketoprofen, and naproxen sodium are all NSAIDs available over-the-counter.

- If you are pregnant, or may become pregnant, you should consult your doctor before using NSAIDs. It is especially important not to use NSAIDs during the last 3 months of pregnancy unless specifically directed to do so by a doctor because it may cause problems in the fetus or complications during delivery.
- Taking the manufacturer's recommended doses of NSAIDs is considered relatively safe for the nursing mother. However, check with your nurse information service or doctor before using this product.
- Do not take NSAIDs if you suffer from asthma, kidney disease, congestive heart failure, diabetes, high blood pressure, heart disease, or if you are scheduled for surgery, without first checking with your doctor.
- Do not use NSAIDs if you are taking a prescription drug to lower high blood pressure; an anticoagulant drug such as warfarin; digoxin; phenytoin; methotrexate; or lithium without first checking with your doctor.
- Do not drink alcohol when taking NSAIDs.
- Do not take NSAIDs for more than 10 days if you have no fever or 3 days if you have a fever, unless prescribed by your doctor.
- Older adults should take lower doses of NSAIDs; check with your nurse information service, doctor, or pharmacist.
- Do not take NSAIDs if you are allergic to aspirin.

Treating Your Child

- Keep all drugs in a locked cabinet out of the reach of children.
- Do not give children under 3 months of age any drugs unless instructed by your doctor.
- If using liquid products for children, do not use the dropper from one bottle to measure the dose from another; some formulations come in different strengths.

Your Symptoms and What to Do About Them

ACNE/PIMPLE

The Problem

You have blackheads; whiteheads; clusters of red, inflamed cysts; or thick, painless lumps below the skin surface on your face and possibly on other parts of your body.

Important Information About Acne and Pimples

The tiny sebaceous glands all over the body produce a skin lubricant called sebum. Puberty, menstruation, pregnancy, other shifts in hormone balance, hereditary factors, or certain medications may trigger the production of too much sebum, which plugs the pores of the skin and produces whiteheads. Skin pigments (not dirt) turn them into blackheads. Normal skin bacteria can cause infection and pus. Pimples result when whiteheads rupture the follicle wall and allow sebum, dead cells, and bacteria to invade the skin. Properly treated, acne is generally harmless and tends to clear up after adolescence. Occasionally, antibiotics or drying preparations are prescribed. Vitamins may also help.

Self-Care Measures

- For relief from acne or pimples:
  - Use benzoyl peroxide preparations for mild cases.
  - Wash your skin gently with a warm washcloth (use a fresh washcloth every day) and soap to remove skin oil (steam may open clogged pores).

Treating Your Child

- Approximately one-third of all infants develop pimples about 3 weeks after birth. They may disappear quickly or last for months. Simply wash your baby's face with mild soap and water; use no other treatment.

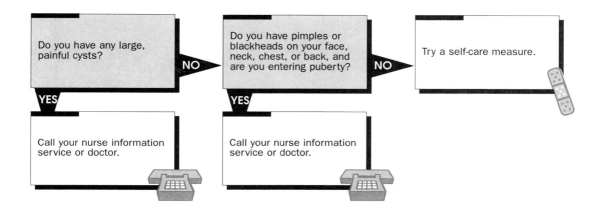

- Wash after exercise or sweating; shampoo often, using a dandruff shampoo if needed.
- Avoid stress (chemicals released by the skin during stressful periods may worsen inflammation).

Prevention

- To help avoid acne or pimples, do not:
  - Use oil-base makeup.
  - Use cortisone preparations.
  - Pick or squeeze lesions.
  - Spend too much time in the sun; or use a sunlamp.
  - Wear tight clothing (the body's pores may become blocked).
  - Touch your face frequently (this may encourage inflammation).

ANKLE PAIN/SWELLING

The Problem

Your ankle is painful, swollen, or bruised.

Causes of Ankle Pain and Swelling

Other Causes

Sprain or strain (*see* page 182)
Rheumatoid arthritis (*see* page 224)
Infectious arthritis
Gout (*see* page 108)
Excess body weight
Dislocation
Heart disease (*see* page 236)
Kidney disease
Nerve damage
Varicose veins
Osteoarthritis (*see* page 224)

Achilles tendinitis. Your ankle has been slowly swelling up over a period of weeks as the tendons became inflamed from overuse.

Fluid or circulation problem. Your ankles have been swollen for more than a day, with no other symptoms. If you've been sitting for a long time (e.g., on a long flight), fluid may "pool" in your feet and ankles. It should go away within 2 days, especially with leg elevation. You may have insufficient veins in your legs or *varicose veins*.

Deep thrombophlebitis (i.e., deep vein thrombosis). Your calf is painful, swollen, and tender when you put weight on your foot; your ankle may be swollen as well. Deep thrombophlebitis is a condition in which a blood clot blocks a vein deep in your leg. A blood clot can be fatal if it breaks away and lodges in a vital organ. You may need blood thinners to break up the clot and prevent additional clots from forming.

Self-Care Measures

- If you have a sprain or strain, try the RICE remedy (*see* page 182).
- For pain and swelling, take aspirin, ibuprofen, or acetaminophen (*see* page 27).
- Ease a strained Achilles tendon by inserting a lift or pad in your shoe heel.
- Get appropriate exercise. Regular use of your legs and feet (e.g., walking, jogging, or using a treadmill) will strengthen your muscles and support tissues around your ankle.
- Soak your feet in cold water for 15 to 20 minutes at a time, several times a day, as soon after the injury as possible.

Treating Your Child

- Don't give aspirin to anyone under 19 years of age! It may cause a rare but serious problem called Reye's syndrome. Instead, use ibuprofen or acetaminophen (*see* page 27) for fever or pain.

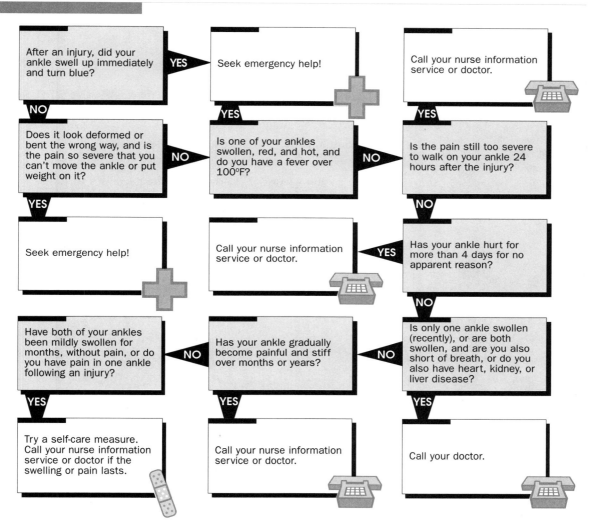

After an injury, did your ankle swell up immediately and turn blue? — **YES** → Seek emergency help!

NO ↓

Does it look deformed or bent the wrong way, and is the pain so severe that you can't move the ankle or put weight on it? — **NO** → Is one of your ankles swollen, red, and hot, and do you have a fever over 100°F? — **NO** → Is the pain still too severe to walk on your ankle 24 hours after the injury?

Call your nurse information service or doctor. (**YES**)

YES ↓ — Seek emergency help!

Is one of your ankles swollen... **YES** ↓ — Call your nurse information service or doctor.

Is the pain still too severe... **NO** ↓

Has your ankle hurt for more than 4 days for no apparent reason? — **YES** → Call your nurse information service or doctor.

NO ↓

Have both of your ankles been mildly swollen for months, without pain, or do you have pain in one ankle following an injury? — **NO** → Has your ankle gradually become painful and stiff over months or years? — **NO** → Is only one ankle swollen (recently), or are both swollen, and are you also short of breath, or do you also have heart, kidney, or liver disease?

YES ↓ — Try a self-care measure. Call your nurse information service or doctor if the swelling or pain lasts.

YES ↓ — Call your nurse information service or doctor.

YES ↓ — Call your doctor.

- Surgical support stockings can help reduce chronic swelling. Ask your nurse information service or doctor for more information.
- After the pain and swelling lessen, gently rotate and bend your ankle several times a day to keep it flexible.

Prevention

- Avoid injuries by wearing the proper shoes: jogging shoes for jogging, tennis shoes for tennis, and so on. Use cushioned inner soles if you are on your feet a lot. Place arch supports in shoes that need them to prevent your feet from rolling inward.

33

APPETITE LOSS

Other Causes

Medication side effect
Depression (*see* page 238)
Common cold (*see* page 176)
Influenza
Infection
Zinc deficiency
Underactive thyroid gland
Alcoholism (*see* page 220)
Anemia (*see* page 90)
Gastritis
Liver disorder
Kidney disorder
Addison's disease
Cancer
Drug use

The Problem

You're simply not hungry; you may have to force yourself to eat.

Causes of Appetite Loss

Aging. You are over 60, and you feel hungry less often. The process of aging can decrease appetite without significant weight loss. As people age, their metabolism slows down and their muscle mass decreases; they don't need as many calories, so their appetite decreases to compensate. In addition, taste sensations and stomach secretions diminish, contributing to appetite loss.

Treating Your Child

- In the absence of other symptoms, a fluctuating appetite is perfectly normal in a child. When children are sick, they generally lose their appetites. This is normal, and forcing them to eat may provoke vomiting.

- Remember that children's stomachs are much smaller than adults', and that appropriate portions for children can be as little as 1/4 to 1/2 of what would satisfy an adult.

- Adults often eat just because they enjoy the experience of eating, but children's appetites are more closely controlled by their bodies' actual energy requirements. Most children have larger appetites when they're in the midst of a growth spurt, but they may eat very little when they're not in a period of active growth. As long as your child is growing normally and does not seem fatigued or sickly, don't worry or try to override the natural appetite-regulating mechanism by forcing your child to eat.

- Most children go through phases in which they seem to be eating only one or two types of food at their meals. There is little danger that a child who eats a limited diet will develop malnutrition. The best way to cope with this is to ignore it; eventually, boredom or curiosity will stimulate your child to accept more foods. Call your nurse information service or doctor only if your child seems fatigued or sickly or is failing to grow at the expected rate. Avoid buying and offering your child unhealthy foods just because she would prefer those foods over more nutritious ones.

- Toddlers may become so attached to sucking on bottles (as a way to deal with boredom, frustration, fatigue, etc.) that they bloat themselves on too much liquid, such as juice or milk, and refuse to eat more nutritious foods. Limit the amount of liquid a child gets from sucking on a bottle or spout cup to 24 ounces a day. If he is really thirsty, he'll take sips from an open cup.

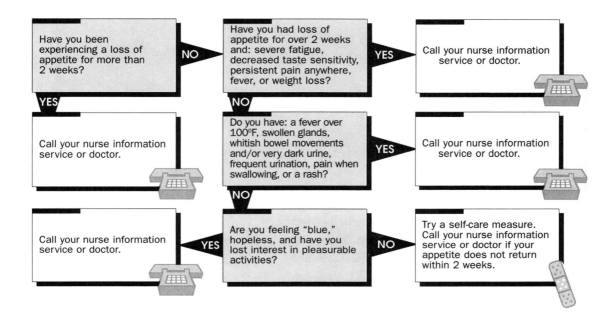

Anorexia nervosa. You eat very little, and you've lost a great deal of weight. You are constantly being told how thin you are, but you don't understand why; you think you are fat. If you're female, you may have stopped having menstrual periods. Anorexia nervosa is a disease that mostly affects women and adolescent girls, causing them to virtually deny the need to eat. Self-care is never sufficient for this disorder, which can be life-threatening if not effectively treated.

Self-Care Measures

- If you're taking one or more medications and you haven't been hungry lately, consult your doctor about a possible change in medication.
- Eat small, frequent, appetizing meals. Eating foods that especially appeal to you is a good way to stimulate your appetite and to get the calories you need.

Prevention

- Take a daily vitamin-and-mineral supplement. Zinc deficiency can cause a loss of appetite by diminishing or altering taste. Over-the-counter supplements can correct this condition.

BACKACHE

The Problem

You have pain and/or stiffness in your upper, middle, or lower back.

Other Causes

Sprain or strain (*see* page 182)
Kidney infection
Scoliosis
Kidney stone (*see* page 204)
Arthritis (*see* page 224)
Prolapsed disk
Osteoporosis (*see* page 250)
Endometriosis
Aortic *aneurysm*
Pneumonia
Heart attack (*see* page 54)
Pelvic inflammatory disease
  (*see* page 208)
Spinal cord damage
Uterine fibroid

Causes of Backache

Poor posture. Your upper back hurts. Poor posture can weaken muscles and strain joints, leading to repeated episodes of pain. Try to stand up straight, and ask your nurse information service or doctor for exercises to increase the flexibility of your back and the strength of your abdominal muscles.

Gallbladder problem. You have pain in your upper right abdomen that spreads into your back, right shoulder, and chest. You may also have fever and chills, nausea or vomiting, abdominal bloating, and heartburn.

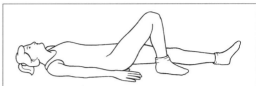

Lie flat on your back on the floor or other hard, flat surface. Bend your knee, keeping your foot flat on the floor.

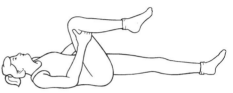

Bring your knee slowly up towards your chest, supporting it with both hands. Hold the position while you count to 10 and then drop your leg gently down to the floor. Repeat with the other leg.

Self-Care Measures

- Complete bed rest is generally not necessary. Activity as tolerated leads to more rapid recovery. When you must get up, do it slowly, by rolling onto your side, swinging your legs to the floor, and pushing off the bed with your arms.

Treating Your Child

- Do not give aspirin to anyone under 19 years of age! It may cause a rare but serious problem called Reye's syndrome. Instead, use ibuprofen or acetaminophen (*see* page 27) for fever or pain.
- If your child complains of back pain after an injury and has difficulty moving her arms or legs, call your nurse information service or doctor immediately.
- Backaches are unusual in children, so if your child complains of pain, call your nurse information service or doctor.

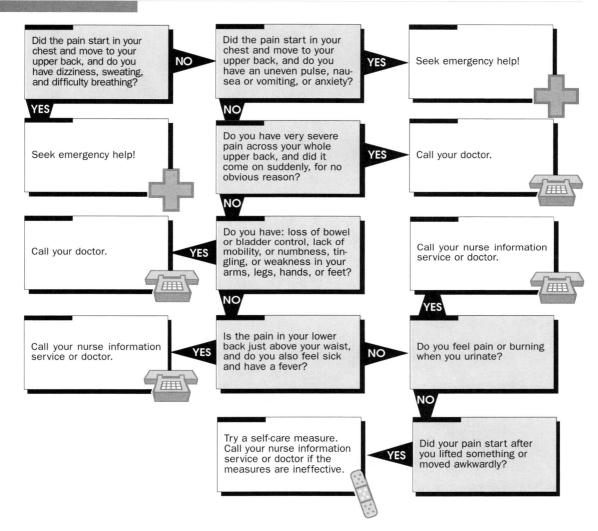

Did the pain start in your chest and move to your upper back, and do you have dizziness, sweating, and difficulty breathing? — **NO**

Did the pain start in your chest and move to your upper back, and do you have an uneven pulse, nausea or vomiting, or anxiety? — **YES** → Seek emergency help!

YES → Seek emergency help!

NO

Do you have very severe pain across your whole upper back, and did it come on suddenly, for no obvious reason? — **YES** → Call your doctor.

NO

Call your doctor. ← **YES** — Do you have: loss of bowel or bladder control, lack of mobility, or numbness, tingling, or weakness in your arms, legs, hands, or feet?

Call your nurse information service or doctor.

NO

Call your nurse information service or doctor. ← **YES** — Is the pain in your lower back just above your waist, and do you also feel sick and have a fever? — **NO** → Do you feel pain or burning when you urinate?

YES (from the nurse information box above)

NO

Try a self-care measure. Call your nurse information service or doctor if the measures are ineffective. ← **YES** — Did your pain start after you lifted something or moved awkwardly?

- When in bed, take the pressure off your lower back by lying on your side with your knees bent and a small pillow between them, or by putting a pillow under your knees when lying on your back.
- Take an over-the-counter medicine containing aspirin, ibuprofen, naproxen sodium, or acetaminophen (*see* page 27).
- If your backache is caused by a muscle injury, apply a cold pack (you can make one by wrapping ice in a towel) for 20 minutes. Sometimes alternating cold

and heat or applying heat alone may be more effective. Then take it off for 20 minutes. Repeat 3 or 4 times.

Prevention

- If you do a lot of lifting, ask your nurse information service or doctor for pointers on how to do it properly (*see* figure, page 246). Wear a corset or special belt to support your back muscles while lifting.
- Sleep on a firm mattress.

BED-WETTING

The Problem

Your child involuntarily urinates during sleep more often than
once a month.

Important Information About Bed-Wetting

It is important to understand that bed-wetting is not the child's fault.
They do not do it deliberately. Most children are embarrassed and
ashamed of wetting their beds and would gladly stop if they could.
Therefore, they need support and encouragement, not punishment and
shame. In the great majority of cases, the causes of bed-wetting in
children are not known; in a small minority of cases, bed-wetting may be
caused by urinary tract infection or diabetes. It is quite common in
children up until the age of 7.

Self-Care Measures

- Buy disposable, absorbent underwear (pull-ups) for your child to wear
  to bed.

Prevention

- Make sure your child urinates before getting into bed at night.
  Decrease his fluid intake for 2 hours before bedtime.

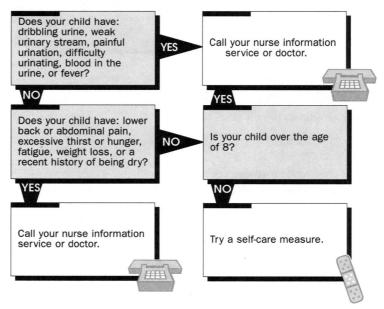

Does your child have: dribbling urine, weak urinary stream, painful urination, difficulty urinating, blood in the urine, or fever?

YES → Call your nurse information service or doctor.

NO ↓

Does your child have: lower back or abdominal pain, excessive thirst or hunger, fatigue, weight loss, or a recent history of being dry?

NO → Is your child over the age of 8?

YES ↓ (from first box)

YES → Call your nurse information service or doctor.

NO → Try a self-care measure.

BITE, ANIMAL/HUMAN

The Problem

You've been bitten by an animal or person. The resulting wound may be superficial (affecting only the top layer of skin) or deep.

Important Information About Bites

For important information about bites, *see* page 64.

Self-Care Measures

- Bites can usually be treated like other cuts or puncture wounds (*see* page 64).

Prevention

- Avoid animals that act strangely, attack without provocation, drool, or "foam at the mouth" — they may have rabies (*see* page 64).

Treating Your Child

- See *Self-Care Measures* and *Prevention* listed here.

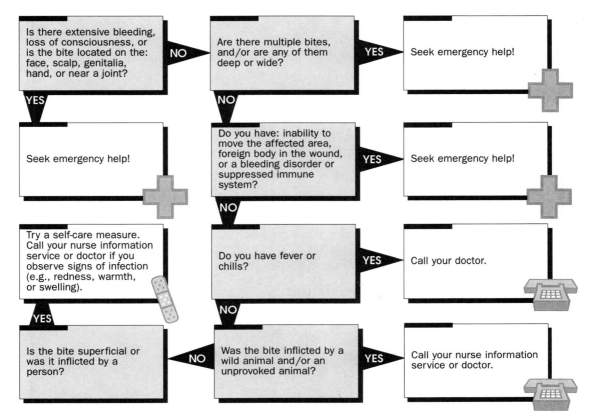

Is there extensive bleeding, loss of consciousness, or is the bite located on the: face, scalp, genitalia, hand, or near a joint?

NO → Are there multiple bites, and/or are any of them deep or wide?

YES → Seek emergency help!

YES (down) → Seek emergency help!

NO (down) → Do you have: inability to move the affected area, foreign body in the wound, or a bleeding disorder or suppressed immune system?

YES → Seek emergency help!

NO (down) → Do you have fever or chills?

YES → Call your doctor.

Try a self-care measure. Call your nurse information service or doctor if you observe signs of infection (e.g., redness, warmth, or swelling).

YES (down, from self-care box) → Is the bite superficial or was it inflicted by a person?

NO (down, from fever box) → Was the bite inflicted by a wild animal and/or an unprovoked animal?

Is the bite superficial or was it inflicted by a person? ← **NO** ← Was the bite inflicted by a wild animal and/or an unprovoked animal?

YES → Call your nurse information service or doctor.

39

BLEEDING

The Problem

Blood is spurting from a cut or wound, and you can't stop it by pressing down onto the wound. You may be bleeding heavily from a minor injury.

Other Causes

Cut (see page 64)
Scrape or abrasion (see page 168)
Anticoagulant therapy
Hormonal disorders
Infection
Radiotherapy
Chemotherapy

Causes of Bleeding

Von Willebrand's disease. You bruise easily, have frequent nosebleeds, bleed heavily from cuts or during menstrual periods, have blood in your urine or stool, and your joints are swollen and painful. Von Willebrand's disease is caused by the lack of a clotting factor in the blood and cannot be prevented. Medications such as aspirin that promote bleeding should not be used. Women with a severe form of the disease may be able to control unusually heavy menstrual bleeding with prescribed oral contraceptives.

Hemophilia. You are a male who has noticed that you bruise and bleed more easily and frequently than most people. Or you have an infant son whose knees and elbows began to bruise and bleed as soon as he started crawling. Hemophilia is an inherited disease in which people lack a specific protein needed for normal clotting. Today there is effective treatment, but you still have to be very careful.

Thrombocytopenia. You have nosebleeds, your cuts bleed for a long time, your periods have become much heavier, and you get a rash of tiny bright and dark red spots wherever your skin is irritated and sometimes even where it's not. This illness, usually resulting from a recent viral infection, medication, or no clear cause, but sometimes associated with leukemia or Hodgkin's disease, is caused by a low level of *platelets* in the blood.

Self-Care Measures

Stop the flow of blood immediately. Follow these steps:

Treating Your Child

See *Self-Care Measures* and *Prevention* listed here.

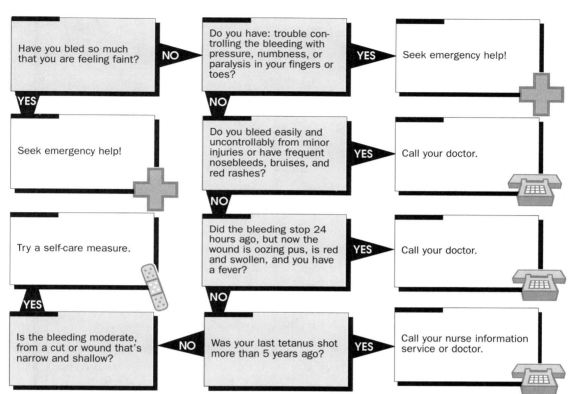

Have you bled so much that you are feeling faint? — **NO** → Do you have: trouble controlling the bleeding with pressure, numbness, or paralysis in your fingers or toes? — **YES** → Seek emergency help!

Have you bled so much that you are feeling faint? — **YES** → Seek emergency help!

Do you have: trouble controlling the bleeding with pressure, numbness, or paralysis in your fingers or toes? — **NO** → Do you bleed easily and uncontrollably from minor injuries or have frequent nosebleeds, bruises, and red rashes? — **YES** → Call your doctor.

Seek emergency help! → Try a self-care measure.

Do you bleed easily and uncontrollably from minor injuries or have frequent nosebleeds, bruises, and red rashes? — **NO** → Did the bleeding stop 24 hours ago, but now the wound is oozing pus, is red and swollen, and you have a fever? — **YES** → Call your doctor.

Try a self-care measure. — **YES** → Is the bleeding moderate, from a cut or wound that's narrow and shallow?

Did the bleeding stop 24 hours ago, but now the wound is oozing pus, is red and swollen, and you have a fever? — **NO** → Was your last tetanus shot more than 5 years ago? — **YES** → Call your nurse information service or doctor.

Is the bleeding moderate, from a cut or wound that's narrow and shallow? — **NO** → Was your last tetanus shot more than 5 years ago?

- Press down firmly and directly over the wound for 5 to 10 minutes, using a clean cloth or gauze pad. Do not use a tourniquet.
- Put on a snug adhesive bandage, or wrap a cloth (firmly but not tightly) around the wound if it's on an arm or leg.
- Elevate the limb or body part that's bleeding.
- If blood oozes through, put another bandage on; don't remove the original, or the bleeding may start again.
- When the bleeding has completely stopped, cleanse the wound (soap and water or 3% hydrogen peroxide). Use "butterfly" bandages to hold the sides together if the wound gapes (*see* page 64).
- Styptic pencils (available over-the-counter) can stop bleeding from small nicks.

- For nosebleeds, sit quietly and press firmly with your thumb and fingers just below the nasal bone to keep the nostrils tightly closed for at least 5 minutes. Do not put your head between your legs or ice on your forehead. If blood continues to drip down the back of your throat, call your nurse information service or doctor.

Prevention

If you are prone to bleeding, take acetaminophen (see page 27), instead of aspirin or ibuprofen, for pain or headaches. Check with your nurse information service or doctor about the use of anticoagulants, especially before surgery.

BLISTER

The Problem

You have a bump on your skin that is tender to the touch and may be swollen with fluid.

Other Causes

Burn (*see* page 52)
Shingles
Contact dermatitis (*see* page 78)

Causes of Blisters

Friction. You've been wearing a pair of shoes that don't quite fit, or a repetitive activity has irritated your skin (playing the guitar, perhaps, or raking the lawn), and now you have a blister. Most blisters are caused by friction—something rubbing against your skin. Self-care is frequently all that is necessary.

Medication. You've started taking a medication within the past couple of days, and now you notice that blisters are forming somewhere—or everywhere—on your body. Sensitivity or allergy to several kinds of medication, including some antibiotics, diuretics, and pain relievers, can cause blisters. Call your nurse information service or doctor and ask whether you need to change medication.

Herpes. You had a tingling or burning before the appearance of watery blisters in the genital area. The blisters fill with pus and become large, painful sores that crust or dry before healing. Herpes simplex is a contagious infection that never leaves once you've been infected.

Self-Care Measures

- If the top of your blister is intact (closed), leave it alone. Cushion it if necessary with a fabric bandage or with adhesive felt or foam.
- If the blister is on your foot, try nonmedicated callus or corn pads to cushion the area, and change your shoes if they don't fit properly.
- If your blister is open and not dirty, fold the skin back over it so that your skin protects the sore area. Then bandage it with a fabric bandage or clean gauze pad.

Treating Your Child
- See *Self-Care Measures* and *Prevention* listed here.

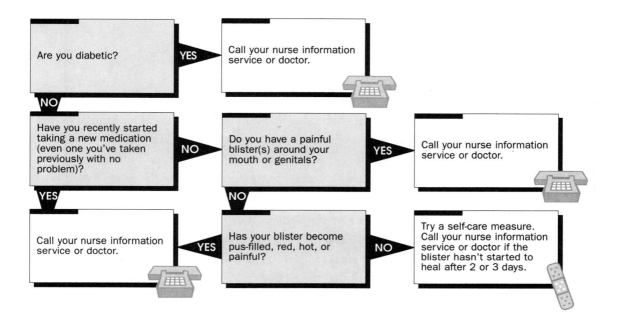

- If your blister is open and dirty, wash the area thoroughly with soap and water, and then bandage it.
- For herpes:
  - Wash the infected area twice daily with soap and water; take a hot bath if you can tolerate it.
  - Apply ice or ice-cold compresses for 5 to 10 minutes at a time.
  - Wear loose cotton clothing.
  - Avoid stress.
  - Try an over-the-counter pain reliever like aspirin, acetaminophen, or ibuprofen (*see* page 27).

- Avoid sexual contact with anyone who has sores on the genitals, anus, or tongue, or who complains of genital tingling or irritation. To prevent infecting others, always use a latex condom for all sexual contact.

Prevention

- Try to protect your skin from sources of friction.
- Wear shoes that fit properly. Break in new boots gradually before going on a long hike.
- Wear heavy gloves for repetitive activities, such as gardening.

BREAST PAIN

The Problem

You have pain in one or both breasts. You may also have swelling and tenderness.

Other Causes

Menopause (*see* page 206)

Causes of Breast Pain

Premenstrual syndrome. Your breasts feel full and painfully tender. A good support bra and other self-care measures may help. Regular breast self-examination will make you familiar with menstrual lumpiness. If you recognize a new or different lump, call your nurse information service or doctor. The best time for breast self-exam is immediately following the end of your period.

Mastitis. You are breast-feeding, your nipples are dry and slightly cracked, and bacteria have produced an infection, making an area of your breast swollen, red, painful or tender, and hot. It is best if you drain the infected breast by nursing more frequently on that side or by using a breast pump. Use hot compresses to massage the tender area while nursing or pumping. You may need antibiotics.

Milk production. Breast discomfort is very common a few days after childbirth. This is usually the result of breast engorgement (swelling) when milk is produced. It is usually relieved by breast-feeding. Hot showers and compresses can help.

Fibrocystic disease. You have lumpy, tender breasts, especially the week before menstruation, or you have several distinct, rounded lumps that move freely inside the breast tissue. The pain can be severe. This condition is more common in older women and can be treated through dietary restrictions, vitamins, hormones, or removal of fluid from cysts.

Self-Care Measures

• If your pain is premenstrual, try nonimpact exercise, such as walking, swimming, or biking. Wear a good support bra, not just

Treating Your Child

• See *Self-Care Measures* and *Prevention* listed here.

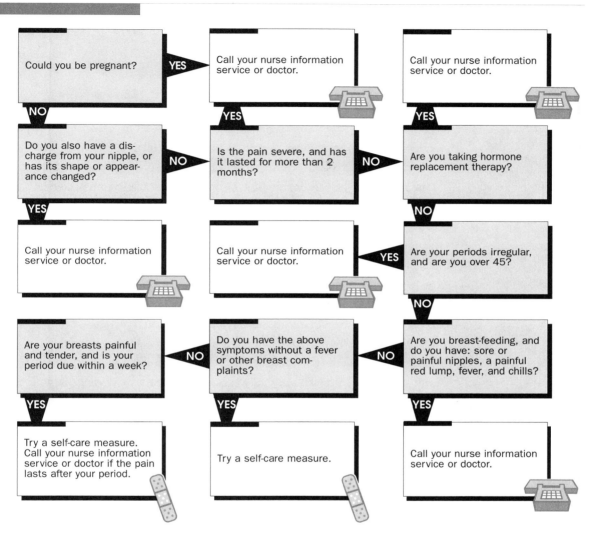

Could you be pregnant? — **YES** → Call your nurse information service or doctor.

NO ↓

Do you also have a discharge from your nipple, or has its shape or appearance changed? — **NO** → Is the pain severe, and has it lasted for more than 2 months? — **YES** → Call your nurse information service or doctor.

YES ↓

Call your nurse information service or doctor.

Is the pain severe... — **NO** → Are you taking hormone replacement therapy? — **YES** → Call your nurse information service or doctor.

NO ↓

Are your periods irregular, and are you over 45? — **YES** → Call your nurse information service or doctor.

NO ↓

Are you breast-feeding, and do you have: sore or painful nipples, a painful red lump, fever, and chills? — **YES** → Call your nurse information service or doctor.

NO → Do you have the above symptoms without a fever or other breast complaints? — **YES** → Try a self-care measure.

NO → Are your breasts painful and tender, and is your period due within a week? — **YES** → Try a self-care measure. Call your nurse information service or doctor if the pain lasts after your period.

while exercising, but at all times, even in bed. Ibuprofen (*see* page 28) may help; so may ice packs.

- Avoid salt, chocolate, coffee, tea, sodas, and other products containing caffeine, including certain cold preparations (read the label). If the discomfort from fluid retention lasts, call your nurse information service or doctor.
- If you have mastitis, acetaminophen (*see* page 27) may help.

Prevention

- To avoid sore or cracked nipples during breast-feeding, make sure the nipple is positioned far back enough in the infant's mouth. Proper positioning and latch-on will resolve this problem.

45

BREATH, BAD

The Problem
Your breath has an offensive odor.

Other Causes

Cigarette smoking
Hiatal hernia (*see* page 118)
Periodontal disease (*see* page 104)
Gingivitis (*see* page 104)
Upper respiratory tract infection
Diabetes (*see* page 240)
Digestive problem
Liver disease
Lung disease
Kidney disease

Causes of Bad Breath

Poor dental hygiene. You have offensive breath, with no other symptoms. You sometimes neglect to brush your teeth twice a day, or you often rush through the task. Inadequate dental hygiene is the most common cause of bad breath. The odor is actually caused by bacteria that live on decaying food particles lodged between your teeth. Self-care is all that's needed to correct this problem, but you should also visit your dentist twice a year for professional cleanings.

Dry mouth. You have bad breath, and you notice that your mouth often feels parched. Saliva contains enzymes that help minimize the bacterial contamination in your mouth; so when your mouth lacks saliva, the bacterial count can shoot up, producing bad breath. It's actually dry mouth that causes the "morning breath" that most adults experience when they awaken from sleep. Certain drugs, including antihistamines and some antidepressants, can also cause bad breath by drying out your mouth.

Tooth decay. You have bad breath along with tooth pain (especially after eating sweet or sour foods), tooth sensitivity to heat and cold, and an unpleasant taste in your mouth. If you have these symptoms and it has been more than 6 months since you've seen a dentist, tooth decay is the probable cause.

Treating Your Child

- Upper respiratory tract infections can cause bad breath in children because they breathe through their mouths; so, if your child's breath has a foul odor, check for other signs of upper respiratory tract infection, such as throat pain.

- A foreign body lodged in a nostril (*see* page 153) can be a cause of bad breath in a young child, especially if you notice drainage from only one side of the nose.

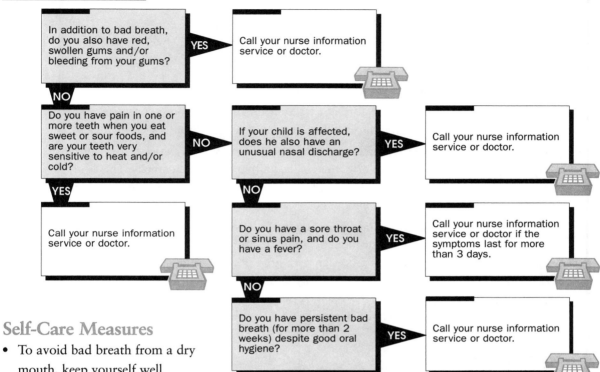

In addition to bad breath, do you also have red, swollen gums and/or bleeding from your gums? **YES** → Call your nurse information service or doctor.

NO ↓

Do you have pain in one or more teeth when you eat sweet or sour foods, and are your teeth very sensitive to heat and/or cold? **NO** → If your child is affected, does he also have an unusual nasal discharge? **YES** → Call your nurse information service or doctor.

YES ↓

Call your nurse information service or doctor.

NO ↓

Do you have a sore throat or sinus pain, and do you have a fever? **YES** → Call your nurse information service or doctor if the symptoms last for more than 3 days.

NO ↓

Do you have persistent bad breath (for more than 2 weeks) despite good oral hygiene? **YES** → Call your nurse information service or doctor.

Self-Care Measures

- To avoid bad breath from a dry mouth, keep yourself well hydrated. Drink 6-8 glasses of water throughout the day.
- Practice good oral hygiene by flossing and brushing your teeth at least twice a day (in the morning and at night before bed). Use a fluoride toothpaste and a soft-bristled toothbrush, as hard bristles can irritate your gums and wear away tooth enamel. Gently brush along the gum line, and do one section of your teeth at a time. The brushing process should take at least 3 minutes; try timing yourself to make sure that you're spending enough time. Rinse thoroughly after brushing; it doesn't make sense to brush the bacteria off your teeth only to let it settle back on.
- Don't forget to brush your tongue. Bacteria and plaque on the tongue are significant sources of bad breath. Brush as far back on the tongue as possible, and gently brush the inside of your cheeks as well.
- Despite all it promises to do for you, the use of mouthwash is not a good idea. Many merely perfume the breath, and the ones that have a high alcohol content can irritate your mouth, which may actually worsen the problem.

Prevention

- Remember to brush twice a day (including your gums, tongue, and the inside of your cheeks) and stay well hydrated.
- Avoid foods that cause bad breath; onions and garlic are the biggest offenders.
- Brushing your teeth or using mouthwash after eating these foods won't help, because the odor actually emanates from your lungs.

BREATHING DIFFICULTY

The Problem

You feel breathless or feel as if you can't get enough air no matter how hard you breathe ("air hunger").

Causes of Breathing Difficulties

Acute respiratory illness. Your breathing is labored or noisy, and you cough and have chills, a fever, and a sore throat.

Hyperventilation. You are under a lot of stress, you start breathing faster, your mouth or hands tingle, and you may feel panicky. This is not dangerous, but it can be frightening. Counseling and instruction in breathing techniques can help.

Chronic or infectious respiratory disease. You are or were a smoker. You've had trouble breathing for some time and it's getting worse, you have a habitual cough with gray or green-yellow *sputum,* or you get winded much more easily than you used to. These symptoms could signal chronic bronchitis (*see* page 232), chronic obstructive pulmonary disease (COPD)(*see* page 232), emphysema (*see* page 232), or lung *cancer.*

Other Causes

Asthma (*see* page 226)
Anxiety or stress
Anaphylaxis
Heart attack (*see* page 54)
Heart disease (*see* page 236)
Anemia (*see* page 90)
Diabetic acidosis
Pneumonia
Diphtheria
Epiglottitis
Obesity (*see* page 248)
Pneumothorax
Sickle cell anemia

Self-Care Measures

- For hyperventilation, scrunch the top of a paper bag closed with one hand, and wiggle a finger of your other hand into the opening to make a small hole. Then slowly breathe in and out of the bag for 5 minutes. Ask your nurse information service or doctor for

Treating Your Child

- You should seek emergency help if your child demonstrates any of the following warning signs and has not been diagnosed as having asthma:
  - Wheezing or breathing loudly enough to be heard 10 feet away, grunting, or making a crowing noise.
  - Running a high fever with a cough.
  - Drooling or refusing to swallow because it hurts to eat or swallow saliva.
  - Flaring nostrils and rapid breathing.
  - Working so hard to breathe that she cannot lie down and rest.
- If your child has asthma, encourage her to engage in physical activity, especially in sports like swimming. You may help to cut down on the number of attacks by identifying and eliminating trigger factors and using preventative medications.

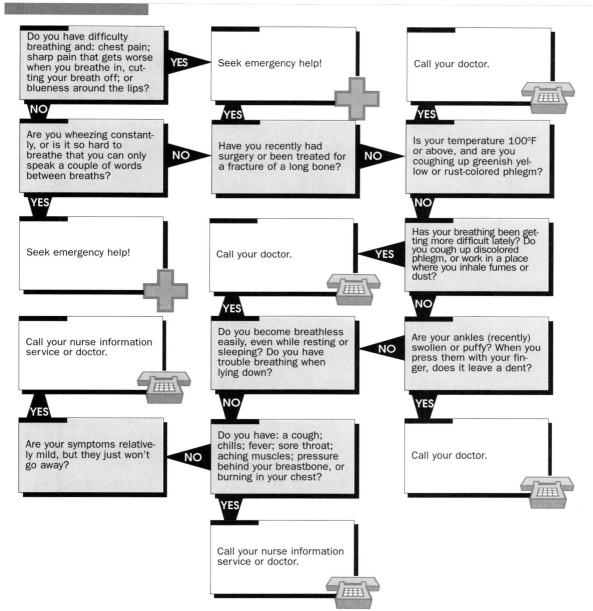

Do you have difficulty breathing and: chest pain; sharp pain that gets worse when you breathe in, cutting your breath off; or blueness around the lips?

YES → Seek emergency help!

NO ↓

Are you wheezing constantly, or is it so hard to breathe that you can only speak a couple of words between breaths?

NO → Have you recently had surgery or been treated for a fracture of a long bone?

YES ↑ Seek emergency help!

YES ↓ Seek emergency help!

Call your nurse information service or doctor.

YES ← Are your symptoms relatively mild, but they just won't go away?

NO ← Do you have: a cough; chills; fever; sore throat; aching muscles; pressure behind your breastbone, or burning in your chest?

YES ↓ Call your nurse information service or doctor.

Call your doctor.

YES ← Do you become breathless easily, even while resting or sleeping? Do you have trouble breathing when lying down?

NO ↓

Is your temperature 100°F or above, and are you coughing up greenish yellow or rust-colored phlegm?

YES ↑ Call your doctor.

NO ↓

Has your breathing been getting more difficult lately? Do you cough up discolored phlegm, or work in a place where you inhale fumes or dust?

YES → Call your doctor.

NO ↓

Are your ankles (recently) swollen or puffy? When you press them with your finger, does it leave a dent?

YES ↓ Call your doctor.

information on special breathing techniques, such as abdominal and purse-lipped breathing, and on exercises to strengthen the *diaphragm* and other breathing muscles.
- If asthma is the cause, *see* page 226.

Prevention
- If you smoke, try to stop.
- If you're overweight and don't exercise, enroll in a fitness program or at least walk 20 minutes, 3 to 4 times a week.
- Swim, especially if you have asthma, both to exercise and to breathe in humid air.

49

BRUISE

The Problem

You have a discolored area on your skin; it is blue, purple, or black at first, but then it gradually fades to yellow. Bruises occur when blood vessels break under your skin and the blood seeps into the surrounding area; the bruise is the spilled blood that is visible under the skin. As the healing process continues, the leaked red blood cells break down and the bruise fades.

Causes of Bruises

Injury. You fell down or hit yourself on something, and now the area is black, blue, or purple. Bruising is a normal reaction to an injury, and the size and shape of the bruise depends on the force of the blow, on the area you injure, and on how easily you bruise. If you injure an area where the skin is thin (e.g., your eye), the bruise and accompanying swelling are likely to be worse. Women generally bruise more easily than men, and everyone bruises more easily after they reach middle age. Bruises are especially common in the elderly on the back of the hands and may appear without any injury to the area. Bruises can almost always be treated with self-care measures.

Iron deficiency anemia. You are very pale, weak, easily fatigued, and you may bruise easily. Iron deficiency anemia is a fairly common condition in which lack of sufficient iron interferes with the red blood cells' ability to carry enough oxygen. This condition is easily treated, under your doctor's supervision, with iron supplements.

Blood platelet disorder. In addition to bruising easily, you notice groups of small, pinpoint-size red specks under your skin; you may also have frequent nosebleeds, gum bleeds with brushing, prolonged menstrual periods, fatigue, and dark stools. Platelets play a vital part in the mechanisms that stop bleeding, so if there is anything wrong with your platelets—if you have too few or if they're not functioning properly—you may bruise easily.

Other Causes

Aplastic anemia
Hemophilia (*see* page 40)
Leukemia
Lymphoma
Lupus erythematosus
Malnutrition
Liver disease
Kidney disease

Treating Your Child

- See *Self-Care Measures* and *Prevention* listed here.

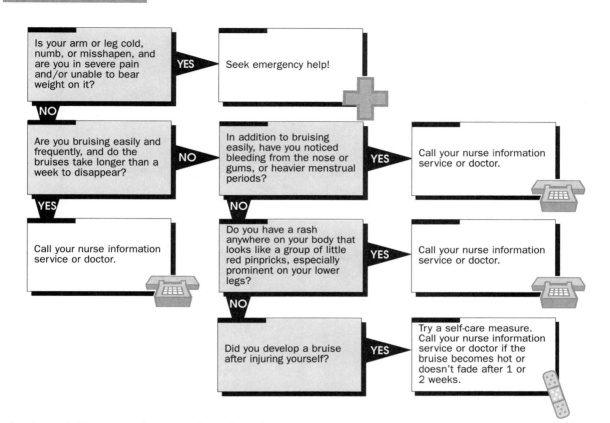

Is your arm or leg cold, numb, or misshapen, and are you in severe pain and/or unable to bear weight on it?

YES → Seek emergency help!

NO

Are you bruising easily and frequently, and do the bruises take longer than a week to disappear?

NO → In addition to bruising easily, have you noticed bleeding from the nose or gums, or heavier menstrual periods?

YES → Call your nurse information service or doctor.

YES → Call your nurse information service or doctor.

NO

Do you have a rash anywhere on your body that looks like a group of little red pinpricks, especially prominent on your lower legs?

YES → Call your nurse information service or doctor.

NO

Did you develop a bruise after injuring yourself?

YES → Try a self-care measure. Call your nurse information service or doctor if the bruise becomes hot or doesn't fade after 1 or 2 weeks.

Blood vessel disease. You bruise easily, and you have frequent nosebleeds and minor bleeding in the mouth or just under the skin that appears as tiny, red pinpoints. You may also have itching, dizziness, night sweats, fatigue, headache, and/or blurred vision.

Self-Care Measures

- Apply ice immediately (using ice cubes wrapped in a washcloth or a bag of frozen vegetables). The ice will help to prevent blood from leaking out of vessels and will minimize black-and-blue marks.

- If the bruise is on an arm or leg, raise the limb above the level of the heart. That will keep blood from pooling in the area and minimize the bruise.

- Don't rub or massage the area. It will only make your bruise worse.

Prevention

- Make sure you're getting enough vitamin C and zinc; both of these nutrients decrease your tendency to bruise. Citrus fruits are good sources of vitamin C, while zinc is found in shellfish, beef, and chicken.

- If you bruise easily, take acetaminophen (*see page 27*) instead of aspirin or ibuprofen, if you need a pain reliever; acetaminophen doesn't affect platelet function.

BURN

The Problem

You have pain from a scald or exposure to fire or chemicals. Your skin is red, blistered, blackened, or white.

Important Information About Burns

Burns can be caused by hot liquids, steam, electric shock, chemicals, and flames. How you treat a burn depends on what caused it and how severe it is. Children and the elderly are at risk for other complications from burns and should seek medical attention early. Burns are classified by degrees:

First-degree burn. Only the outer layer of skin is burned. Skin is red and tender but is not blistering. First-degree burns are not usually serious.

Second-degree burn. You have a severe burn or scald caused by hot liquid, flash from gasoline or other flammable liquids, or a fire. Your burn is painful and swollen, with blisters and a weepy, watery surface. With proper self-care, it should feel better in a day or two and heal within a week.

Third-degree burn. Your burn is severe, deep, and possibly exposes underlying flesh, and your skin is charred or whitened. If your nerves have been burned, you may feel pain around the edges of the burn, but not right on it. Third-degree burns are caused by electrical shocks, clothing on fire, severe gasoline fires, or any intense or prolonged exposure to flames.

Self-Care Measures

- Third-degree burns: If you're waiting for an ambulance, soak the burned area in cold water just long enough to lower the temperature a little. Then wrap the wound or the entire body in a clean bandage or sheet. Don't try to remove any clothing. Don't apply any medication.
- Second-degree burns: Small second-degree burns can be cooled with water, then gently washed with soap and rinsed, sprayed with antiseptic, and lightly covered.

Treating Your Child
- See *Self-Care Measures* listed here and preventative measures on page 22.

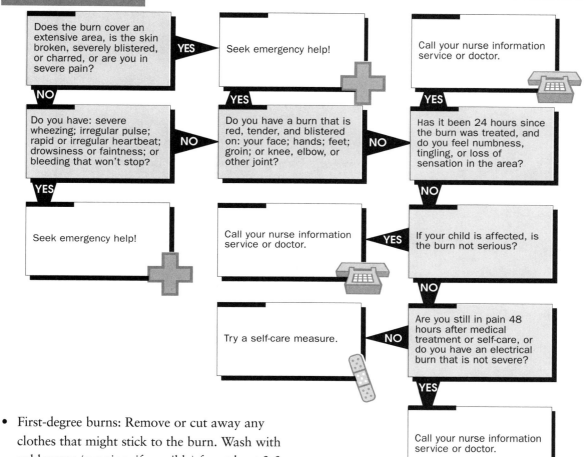

Does the burn cover an extensive area, is the skin broken, severely blistered, or charred, or are you in severe pain?

YES → Seek emergency help!

NO ↓

Do you have: severe wheezing; irregular pulse; rapid or irregular heartbeat; drowsiness or faintness; or bleeding that won't stop?

YES ↓

Seek emergency help!

NO → Do you have a burn that is red, tender, and blistered on: your face; hands; feet; groin; or knee, elbow, or other joint?

YES ↓

Call your nurse information service or doctor.

NO → Has it been 24 hours since the burn was treated, and do you feel numbness, tingling, or loss of sensation in the area?

Call your nurse information service or doctor.

YES ↑

NO ↓

If your child is affected, is the burn not serious?

YES → Call your nurse information service or doctor.

NO ↓

Are you still in pain 48 hours after medical treatment or self-care, or do you have an electrical burn that is not severe?

NO → Try a self-care measure.

YES ↓

Call your nurse information service or doctor.

- First-degree burns: Remove or cut away any clothes that might stick to the burn. Wash with cold water (running, if possible) for at least 2-3 minutes. Then cover with a clean, dry gauze or cloth bandage. Don't use cotton. Don't apply any ointment or medication. Don't use local anesthetic sprays or creams; they can delay healing. Do take aspirin (if you are age 19 or older) or another nonprescription anti-inflammatory medication (e.g., ibuprofen [*see* page 28]); it will help to relieve the pain and also reduces inflammation.
- All burns: After immediate first aid, elevate the burned body part, if possible. While your burn is healing, keep dressings clean, and watch for any sign of redness or swelling, which may mean infection. Don't break any blisters. New skin may dry and crack; try a basic moisturizing cream.
- A *tetanus* shot is necessary if skin is broken and your last tetanus shot was more than 5 years ago.

Prevention
- Don't smoke in bed.
- Install smoke alarms as recommended.
- Don't pour gasoline, kerosene, or lighter fluid on a tick.
- For household fire-prevention measures, *see* page 21.

CHEST PAIN

The Problem

Your chest hurts. The pain may be crushing, burning, dull and pressing, or sharp and stabbing.

Causes of Chest Pain

Other Causes

Anxiety or stress
Heartburn (*see* page 18)
Sprain or strain (*see* page 182)
Respiratory infection
Asthma (*see* page 226)
Hiatal hernia (*see* page 118)
Ulcer
Shingles
Gallbladder problem
Broken rib
Lung *cancer*
Blood clot in the lung
Collapsed lung
Pleurisy

Angina. Part of the heart is not getting enough oxygen. You feel a squeezing pressure, heaviness, or mild ache in the chest. The pain typically occurs when you're active but decreases when you rest. As is the case with heart attacks, this is usually seen in men over 40, post-menopausal women, and people who smoke, have high blood pressure (*see* page 244), diabetes (*see* page 240), or a high cholesterol level.

Heart attack. The blood supply to part of the heart is blocked and part of this muscle dies. Symptoms include severe, crushing pain in the center of the chest that may spread to the arm, shoulder, or jaw; sweating; shortness of breath; and sometimes nausea/vomiting. You may feel faint, dizzy, or very anxious.

Self-Care Measures

- If anxiety/stress is the cause, *see* page 190.

Treating Your Child

- Don't give aspirin to anyone under 19 years of age! It may cause a rare but serious problem called Reye's syndrome. Instead, use ibuprofen or acetaminophen (*see* page 27) for fever or pain.
- Chest pain in children is unlikely to be due to heart problems, unless the child is known to have a heart disorder.
- In early adolescence, sharp chest pain, lasting only a few seconds and occurring at rest, is common and usually of no concern. This type of chest pain typically gets worse with moving the chest wall, such as with

deep breathing, or is located where the rib and breast bones come together. However, if your child's chest pain is brought on by exercise, call your nurse information service or doctor.
- If your child injures his chest while playing, try to get him to rest. If the pain or difficulty breathing lasts for more than several hours, call your nurse information service or doctor.
- Chest pain or light-headedness occurring only with exercise could indicate a rare heart problem.

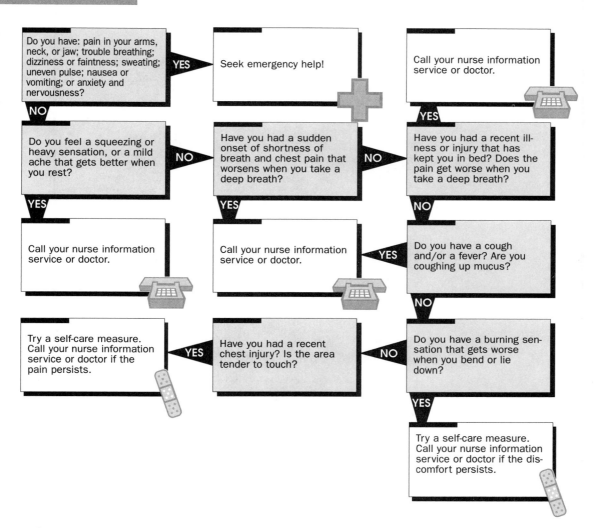

Do you have: pain in your arms, neck, or jaw; trouble breathing; dizziness or faintness; sweating; uneven pulse; nausea or vomiting; or anxiety and nervousness?

YES → Seek emergency help!

NO ↓

Do you feel a squeezing or heavy sensation, or a mild ache that gets better when you rest?

NO → Have you had a sudden onset of shortness of breath and chest pain that worsens when you take a deep breath?

YES → Call your nurse information service or doctor.

YES ↓

Call your nurse information service or doctor.

YES → Call your nurse information service or doctor.

Have you had a recent illness or injury that has kept you in bed? Does the pain get worse when you take a deep breath?

NO ↓

Do you have a cough and/or a fever? Are you coughing up mucus?

YES → Call your nurse information service or doctor.

NO ↓

Try a self-care measure. Call your nurse information service or doctor if the pain persists.

YES ← Have you had a recent chest injury? Is the area tender to touch?

NO ← Do you have a burning sensation that gets worse when you bend or lie down?

YES ↓

Try a self-care measure. Call your nurse information service or doctor if the discomfort persists.

- To relieve angina, try resting in a chair. If you've had angina before and have been given medicine, take the medicine.
- If heartburn is the cause, *see* page 118.
- If a sprain or strain is the cause, *see* page 182.
- If you have an infection, your chest pain may not go away until the infection is treated. Cough medicine may help (as long as you're not coughing up mucus). A cool-mist humidifier will moisten the air and may provide relief.

Prevention

- To avoid a sprain or strain, *see* page 183.
- For a healthy heart: exercise regularly; eat a balanced, low-fat diet; don't smoke.
- To avoid heartburn, *see* page 118.

CONFUSION/FORGETFULNESS

The Problem

A friend or family member suddenly, or over a long period of time, is having trouble remembering things; he may not know where he is, what day it is, or who he is.

Other Causes

Fever (*see* page 94)
Stroke (*see* page 258)
Drug or alcohol use
Malnutrition/vitamin deficiency
Diabetes (*see* page 240)
Hypothermia
Depression (*see* page 238)
Hypoglycemia
Brain tumor
Encephalitis
Syphilis
Hydrocephalus

Causes of Confusion and Forgetfulness

Injury. A blow to the head can cause confusion. This may resolve, but the person should be observed. If confusion or disorientation continues for some time after the injury, there may be bleeding inside the skull, which is serious and requires medical attention.

Transient ischemic attack. The person is confused and forgetful and is also experiencing numbness, tingling, loss of movement in the arms or legs, blurred vision, and difficulty speaking. There may have been a brief interruption in the brain's blood supply, which could be a sign of arterial disease.

Dementia. The person is probably over 65, and his confusion and forgetfulness are accompanied by loss of concern about cleanliness and appearance, the inability to remember what just happened, and changes in personality (such as agitation and irritability). He may be depressed and/or undernourished, or he may have dementia. Although rare, dementia may occur in younger people.

Self-Care Measures

If confusion and/or forgetfulness occur there are no effective self-care measures. Look at the symptom chart to help you decide whether to seek emergency help or call your nurse information service or doctor.

- If fever is the cause, *see* page 95.
- If the person has missed a meal and is diabetic, dried fruit or orange juice may help. Ask the doctor to suggest other snack ideas.

Treating Your Child
- See *Self-Care Measures* and *Prevention* listed here.

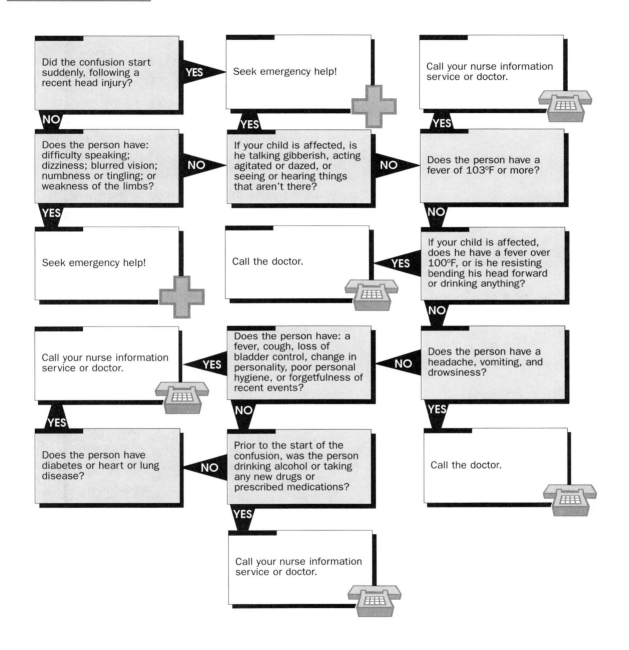

Did the confusion start suddenly, following a recent head injury?

YES → Seek emergency help!

NO ↓

Does the person have: difficulty speaking; dizziness; blurred vision; numbness or tingling; or weakness of the limbs?

YES ↓ Seek emergency help!

NO → If your child is affected, is he talking gibberish, acting agitated or dazed, or seeing or hearing things that aren't there?

YES → Call your nurse information service or doctor.

YES → Call the doctor.

NO → Does the person have a fever of 103°F or more?

YES → Call your nurse information service or doctor.

NO → If your child is affected, does he have a fever over 100°F, or is he resisting bending his head forward or drinking anything?

YES → Call the doctor.

NO ↓

Does the person have: a fever, cough, loss of bladder control, change in personality, poor personal hygiene, or forgetfulness of recent events?

YES → Call your nurse information service or doctor.

NO → Does the person have a headache, vomiting, and drowsiness?

YES → Call the doctor.

NO ↓

Prior to the start of the confusion, was the person drinking alcohol or taking any new drugs or prescribed medications?

YES ← Does the person have diabetes or heart or lung disease?

YES → Call your nurse information service or doctor.

YES ↓ Call your nurse information service or doctor.

Prevention

- Use of over-the-counter medications should be avoided.

- Take steps to get help for drug or alcohol abusers.

CONSTIPATION

The Problem

Your bowel movements are infrequent (i.e., fewer than 3 a week), and the feces are hard, and difficult or uncomfortable to pass.

Other Causes

Inadequate exercise
Overuse of laxatives
Medication side effect
Depression (*see* page 238)
Irritable bowel syndrome
  (see page 186)
Hypothyroidism (*see* page 127)
Hypercalcemia
Kidney failure
Backache (*see* page 36)
Cancer
Appendicitis
Diverticulitis
Pelvic inflammatory disease
  (see page 208)
Peritonitis

Causes of Constipation

Insufficient fluid and fiber intake. Your bowel movements are infrequent, and the feces are dry, small, and difficult to pass. Not getting enough fluid and fiber in your diet is by far the most frequent cause of constipation. Fiber is the nondigestible bulk found in whole grains, fruits, and vegetables. It acts like a sponge in the intestines, drawing in water and making the stool softer. It also keeps your bowel movements regular. However, in order for fiber to draw fluid into your bowel, you must first have enough fluid in your body.

Self-Care Measures

Try a few of the following in combination:

- Set aside a regular time each day for bowel movements; the best time is often within 1 hour after breakfast. Don't hurry; sit for at

Treating Your Child

- Some parents are overly concerned about their child's bowel movements. Like adults, children do not have to have a bowel movement every day or even every other day. Don't suspect constipation unless your child is having difficulty or pain when attempting to have a bowel movement; is complaining of discomfort in the anal area; or is passing hard, dry stools fewer than 3 times a week.
- Children who are new to toilet training or who have been toilet trained recently sometimes "hold their stool," resisting the urge to have a bowel movement. If you suspect this problem in your child, you can help by adopting a more relaxed attitude toward toilet training. Let your child know that it's fine to wear diapers for bowel movements and his "big boy pants" the rest of the time. He can then decide when he's ready to give up diapers altogether.
- Many months of constipation and "stool holding" can lead to a condition in which a child is unaware that he is soiling his pants. It is important to get professional help if this occurs, and ideally before it develops.

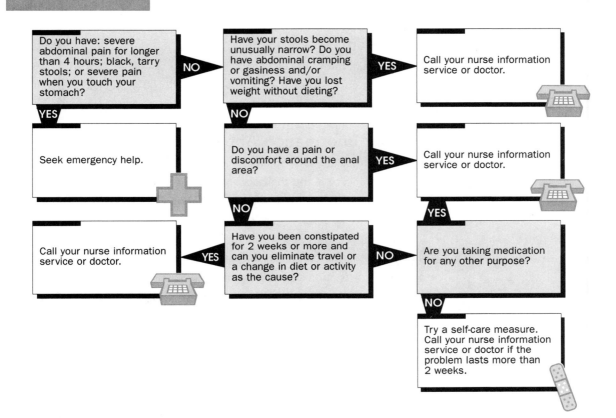

least 10 minutes, whether or not you actually have a bowel movement.

- Try drinking a cup of hot coffee, tea, or water in the morning.
- Include fruits, vegetables, legumes, and bran or other whole-grain cereals in your diet.
- Drink at least 6 to 8 glasses of water a day. Avoid too much caffeine or alcohol, which can be dehydrating.
- Increase your physical activity. Brisk walking, aerobic dance, and jogging can increase your bowel's activity.
- Add an over-the-counter fiber supplement to your diet. Start with 5 grams (i.e., a teaspoon) and increase the dose as tolerated. Be sure to

take it with enough fluid, or you could end up more constipated than before.

- Check your multivitamin supplement. Too much iron intake can cause constipation.
- For occasional constipation, you might want to try an over-the-counter stool softener or an enema; these products are only for occasional use!

Prevention

- Eating a well-balanced, high-fiber diet, drinking plenty of fluids each day, and exercising regularly are by far the best ways to prevent constipation.

CORN/CALLUS

The Problem

You have a small bump of thickened skin on top of one of your toe joints—that's a corn. You have a thickened, hard, rough, yellowish patch of skin on the bottom of your foot—that's a callus.

Important Information About Corns and Calluses

Corns and calluses are very much alike; the primary differences between them are their location and their size. Corns are small and roundish, and they form on the bony area on top of the toe joints and between the toes. Calluses are larger and flatter, and can appear on any part of the body that is repeatedly subjected to pressure and friction: the balls or heels of your feet, the palms of your hands, or your knees. The formation of corns and calluses is the body's protective response to constant pressure or repeated friction. They are very common and usually go away when the pressure/friction is removed, rarely causing serious problems.

Self-Care Measures

If your corn or callus is not causing you discomfort, no action is required. However, if it is bothering you, there are several measures you can take. (Note: If you are a diabetic [*see* page 240] or have *circulatory problems*, do not use self-care).

- Wear only comfortable footwear that fits properly. Remember that your feet tend to enlarge (especially in width) as you get older. Don't assume that your shoe size is the same now as it was in the past; have a professional measure your feet.

Treating Your Child
- See *Self-Care Measures* and *Prevention* listed here.

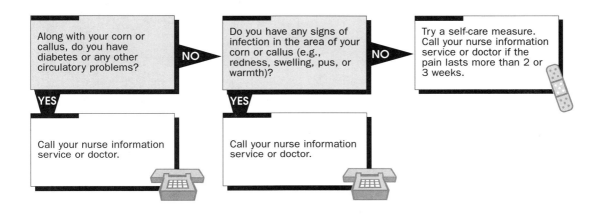

- Soak the affected area in warm, soapy water every day for at least 5 minutes. Then, use a pumice stone or callus file (available in drugstores), or a rough towel to gently rub away the outer layer of thickened skin.
- Many podiatrists (i.e., foot specialists) warn against the use of over-the-counter, acid-based corn and callus removers, because they can cause infection. If you do decide to use one, follow the package directions carefully.
- Ointments containing salicylic acid should not be applied to the affected area.
- Apply a doughnut-shaped piece of felt or moleskin (available in drugstores and supermarkets) to the corn or callus for relief.

Prevention
- Wear comfortable shoes that fit properly to avoid constant pressure and friction, the most common causes of corns and calluses, on the feet.
- To avoid calluses on the hands, work gloves should be worn when performing heavy manual work.

COUGH

The Problem

You have a cough, which is the body's reflex to an irritation in the sinuses, throat, breathing tubes, or lungs. You have either a productive cough, which brings up mucus, or a nonproductive cough, which is dry and hacking.

Other Causes

Heartburn (*see* page 118)
Common cold (*see* page 176)
Asthma (*see* page 226)
Pertussis
Croup
Anaphylaxis
Aneurysm
Lung *cancer*
Collapsed lung
Tuberculosis

Causes of Cough

Cigarette smoking. Your cough may be nonproductive or productive and gagging, and it is worse when you get up in the morning or after smoking. Smoker's cough is caused by the many poisonous chemicals in cigarette smoke, and the only way to get rid of it is to stop smoking (*see* page 24).

Respiratory infection. You have a productive cough and fever (102°F or higher). You are extremely tired, your muscles ache, and you feel too sick to go about your normal daily activities. Coughing up white mucus is usually a sign of a viral infection, which needs to run its course, but you can relieve the symptoms with self-care measures. Green or rust-colored mucus is often a sign of a bacterial infection, which may require an antibiotic.

Treating Your Child

- Don't give aspirin to anyone under 19 years of age! It may cause a rare but serious problem called Reye's syndrome. Instead, use ibuprofen or acetaminophen (*see* page 27) for fever or pain.
- If your child suddenly starts coughing sharply and doesn't have a cold, he or she may have a piece of food or other small object lodged in the windpipe. Seek emergency help!
- Although congestion is common in infants, a persistent cough is unusual in very young infants. If a child under 3 months develops a cough, call your nurse information service or doctor.
- A cough that sounds like a seal's bark, is accompanied by hoarseness, and is worse at night may be croup, an inflammation of the air passages that is common in children. Expose your child to humid air: take him into the bathroom, close the door, stand outside the bathtub, and turn the shower on hot, full blast. If that doesn't help, call your nurse information service or doctor.

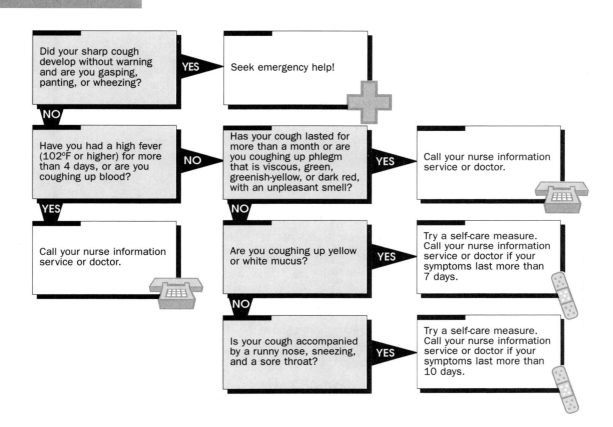

Did your sharp cough develop without warning and are you gasping, panting, or wheezing? **YES** → Seek emergency help!

NO ↓

Have you had a high fever (102°F or higher) for more than 4 days, or are you coughing up blood? **NO** → Has your cough lasted for more than a month or are you coughing up phlegm that is viscous, green, greenish-yellow, or dark red, with an unpleasant smell? **YES** → Call your nurse information service or doctor.

YES ↓

Call your nurse information service or doctor.

NO ↓ (from phlegm question)

Are you coughing up yellow or white mucus? **YES** → Try a self-care measure. Call your nurse information service or doctor if your symptoms last more than 7 days.

NO ↓

Is your cough accompanied by a runny nose, sneezing, and a sore throat? **YES** → Try a self-care measure. Call your nurse information service or doctor if your symptoms last more than 10 days.

Self-Care Measures

- If your cough is productive, don't try to suppress it except at nighttime to allow sleep. Use a cool-mist vaporizer, or take a hot shower to thin the mucus and make it easier to cough up. Try an over-the-counter expectorant cough medicine (look for guaifenesin as an ingredient, but do not use guaifenesin if you have a persistent or chronic cough with large amounts of mucus or an asthma-related cough). Drink plenty of liquids.

- If your cough is nonproductive, try throat lozenges, hard candies, or an over-the-counter cough suppressant (look for the ingredient dextromethorphan, but do not use dextromethorphan if you are taking a monoamine oxidase inhibitor [MAOI] unless directed to by your doctor). You can also try honey mixed with hot water, tea, or lemon juice.

- If a postnasal drip is irritating the back of your throat and causing your cough, over-the-counter decongestants or antihistamines can help dry up the mucus.

- If a common cold is the cause, *see* page 176.

Prevention

- If your cough is caused by smoking, it may be an indicator of far more serious problems to come. Try to quit, and avoid exposure to second-hand smoke (*see* page 24).

CUT

The Problem

Your skin or flesh has been sliced open.

Important Information About Cuts

Most cuts will heal with simple self-care. However, if the cut has affected a muscle, tendon, ligament, nerve, or joint, or if it is gaping, you may need medical care. A *tetanus* shot is necessary if skin is broken and your last tetanus shot was more than 5 years ago (for dirty wounds) or 10 years ago (for clean wounds).

If you've been bitten by an animal and the bite broke the skin, there is a remote chance that you could have been infected with rabies, a viral disease that attacks the central nervous system of mammals. If you've been bitten by someone's pet, it's highly unlikely that you've been infected, but since rabies can be extremely serious, even fatal, check with the owner to see if the animal has had all the necessary immunizations. If you've been bitten by a wild animal, report the bite to your nurse information service, the local health authority, or animal control agency, even if the animal doesn't show the classic signs of active rabies, "foaming at the mouth" or acting aggressively. If possible, bring the animal in to be checked to see if it is rabid. You may need to get a rabies vaccine and/or antirabies serum. *See* symptoms chart on page 39.

Bites inflicted by people can be a source of infection, but bites inflicted by children are less likely to become infected than bites by adults. Call your nurse information service or doctor if there is a possibility that the biter has hepatitis B or is HIV positive, or if the bite is the result of abuse.

Self-Care Measures

- For a cut:
  - Rinse the cut with cold water. Wash it thoroughly with soap and water or 3% hydrogen peroxide, and rinse again. Remove dirt, glass, or any other foreign material with tweezers soaked in alcohol; however, if the material is deeply embedded, seek medical care.
  - If the cut is bleeding, apply a pressure bandage, or hold a gauze pad tightly against it. Close a gaping cut with a butterfly bandage (*see* figures). If the wound is more than 3 or 4 millimeters deep and

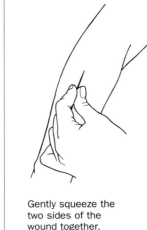

Gently squeeze the two sides of the wound together.

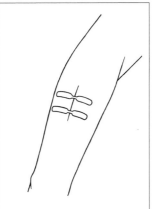

Secure the butterfly bandages every 1/2 inch.

Treating Your Child

- See *Self-Care Measures* and *Prevention* listed here.

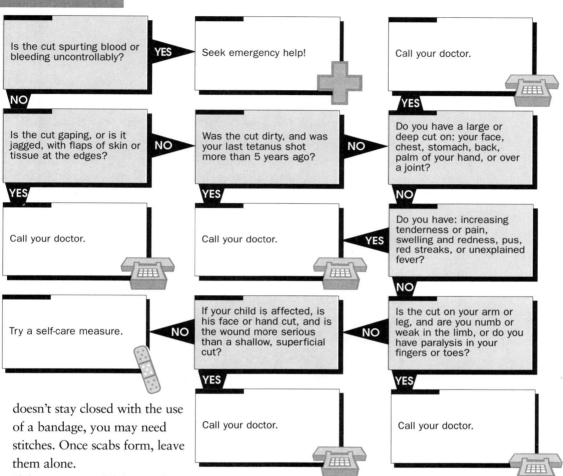

Is the cut spurting blood or bleeding uncontrollably? **YES** → Seek emergency help!

NO ↓

Is the cut gaping, or is it jagged, with flaps of skin or tissue at the edges? **NO** → Was the cut dirty, and was your last tetanus shot more than 5 years ago? **NO** → Do you have a large or deep cut on: your face, chest, stomach, back, palm of your hand, or over a joint?

YES Call your doctor.

YES ↓

Call your doctor.

YES ↓

Call your doctor.

NO ↓

Do you have: increasing tenderness or pain, swelling and redness, pus, red streaks, or unexplained fever? **YES** → Call your doctor.

NO ↓

Try a self-care measure. ← **NO** If your child is affected, is his face or hand cut, and is the wound more serious than a shallow, superficial cut? ← **NO** Is the cut on your arm or leg, and are you numb or weak in the limb, or do you have paralysis in your fingers or toes?

YES ↓

Call your doctor.

YES ↓

Call your doctor.

doesn't stay closed with the use of a bandage, you may need stitches. Once scabs form, leave them alone.

– If the cut is painful (but without signs of infection—redness, swelling, pus), take aspirin, ibuprofen, or acetaminophen (*see* page 27).

• For a puncture wound:
  – Let the wound bleed freely unless there is a great deal of blood loss or blood is spurting from the wound. In that case, apply direct pressure and call your nurse information service or doctor.
  – If the object that caused the puncture is still in the wound, take it out with clean tweezers if you can do so without causing more injury. (Soak the tweezers in alcohol for 20 minutes to clean them.)

– Clean the wound with warm water and soap. Do not cover the wound with a bandage unless it is likely to get dirty.
– Soak the wound in warm, soapy water 2 to 3 times a day for 4 to 5 days. This will keep the wound open so that germs can drain from it.

Prevention

• Exercise care when using sharp tools or kitchen implements. Store them safely, never jumbled together in a drawer. Never leave sharp kitchen implements in a sink full of water.
• Wear heavy gloves when doing construction or repair work around the home.

DANDRUFF

The Problem

Your scalp sheds white flakes.

Other Causes

Contact dermatitis (*see* page 178)

Causes of Dandruff

Seborrheic dermatitis. You have the typical very small snowflakes on your shoulders, with no other symptoms. Or you may have heavy scaling and dandruff flakes around your eyebrows, nose, behind your ears, even under your arms and in the genital areas. There may be redness, crusting, and oozing. The cause is not known for certain but is probably due to a type of fungal infection and is associated with excessive oiliness, and often made worse by physical or emotional stress and by extremely hot, humid weather or very dry cold air. Self-care remedies are usually effective.

Psoriasis. You started with dandruff, but now you have *plaques*, patches of raised, red bumps covered with white, flaking scales on your scalp, knees, elbows, or buttocks. The patches may be itchy or painful. You may also have loosened, discolored nails, and joint pain and stiffness.

Fungal infection. You have itchy, flaking, red or grayish patches on your scalp. You may also have some hair loss. Fungal infections are caused by microscopic organisms. Attacks can range from mild to severe. Poor hygiene is usually the cause. Over-the-counter or prescription medication is sometimes necessary.

Treating Your Child

- Cradle cap is very common in babies, and it can be stubborn to remove. Apply some baby oil (petroleum jelly is too difficult to wash out later) a few minutes before you give the baby a bath, then very gently scrub off the scales with a soft brush made for this purpose. Be careful not to rub too hard as this can cause further irritation. Use a fine-tooth baby comb to remove the remaining scales, then follow up with shampoo to remove the oil. You can try a gentle anti-dandruff shampoo for particularly stubborn cases.

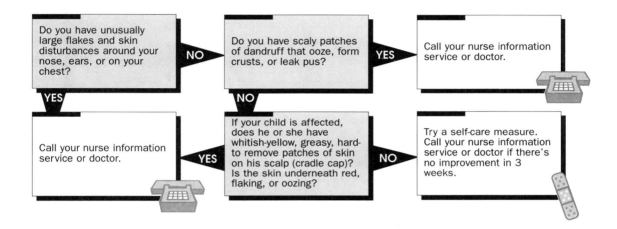

Do you have unusually large flakes and skin disturbances around your nose, ears, or on your chest?

NO → Do you have scaly patches of dandruff that ooze, form crusts, or leak pus?

YES → Call your nurse information service or doctor.

YES ↓

Call your nurse information service or doctor.

NO ↓

If your child is affected, does he or she have whitish-yellow, greasy, hard-to remove patches of skin on his scalp (cradle cap)? Is the skin underneath red, flaking, or oozing?

YES ← Call your nurse information service or doctor.

NO → Try a self-care measure. Call your nurse information service or doctor if there's no improvement in 3 weeks.

Self-Care Measures

- Shampoo daily with a prescription or over-the-counter dandruff shampoo containing sulfur, salicylic acid, selenium, or tar. Follow instructions carefully, being sure to rinse thoroughly. A conditioner may help.

Prevention

- Use dandruff shampoo occasionally, between uses of a regular shampoo. Try using different regular shampoos, alternating days or switching every few days.

DIARRHEA

The Problem

You are having unusually watery and frequent bowel movements; they may be preceded by gas and abdominal cramping.

Causes of Diarrhea

Other Causes

Medication side effect
Irritable bowel syndrome
    (*see* page 186)
Ulcerative colitis
Crohn's disease
Parasitic infection
Alcohol use
Food poisoning (*see* page 148)
Food *allergy*
Cancer
Nutrient malabsorption
    (*see* page 214)

Infection. You have had several episodes of diarrhea, and you also feel sick; you may be vomiting as well. Diarrhea is a common sign of a gastrointestinal infection. These infections can be caused by viruses or bacteria picked up in food or drinking water, or they may be viral and not related to food. In either case, the diarrhea is the body's way of clearing the infection from the intestine. Therefore, it is usually best to let the diarrhea run its course, while keeping yourself well hydrated. Certain gastrointestinal infections require antibiotics.

Lactose intolerance. You've recently eaten ice cream or some other dairy product, and now you have diarrhea. Many adults lack lactase, an enzyme needed to properly digest lactose, which is the sugar in dairy products. As a result, fluid builds up in the intestine, and diarrhea results.

Self-Care Measures

- For the first 24 to 48 hours of severe diarrhea, avoid all solid foods, taking clear liquids only. Dehydration is always a danger with diarrhea, so make

Treating Your Child

- Short-term diarrhea in children is unlikely to have a serious cause or to present any health risk as long as you ensure that your child drinks plenty of fluids while the diarrhea lasts. If dehydration is a problem, *see* page 195. Many children develop diarrhea from drinking juice (especially apple juice) or milk.
- Breast-fed babies normally have frequent, watery stools (i.e., about the consistency of cream soup), so it may be difficult to tell whether they are having diarrhea. Call your nurse information service or doctor if the stools have a foul odor, or if your baby is feeding poorly or acting sick.
- "Toddler's diarrhea" may be the cause if your child's stools are foul-smelling and runny, and the diarrhea lasts for several days. As long as your child remains active, appears healthy, does not have a fever, and stays well hydrated, you need not be concerned. If the diarrhea lasts more than 3 to 4 days, call your nurse information service or doctor.

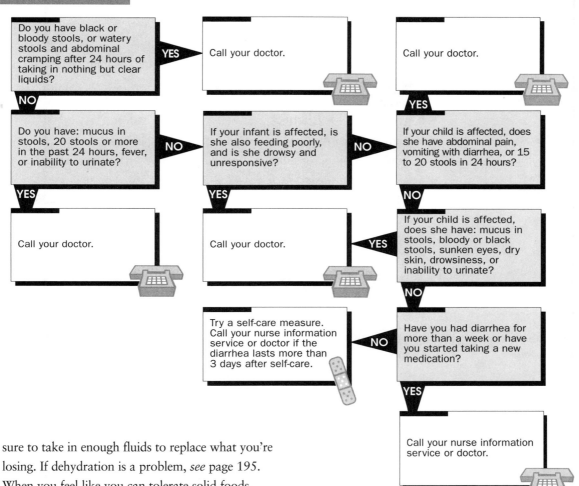

Do you have black or bloody stools, or watery stools and abdominal cramping after 24 hours of taking in nothing but clear liquids?

YES → Call your doctor.

NO

Do you have: mucus in stools, 20 stools or more in the past 24 hours, fever, or inability to urinate?

NO → If your infant is affected, is she also feeding poorly, and is she drowsy and unresponsive?

YES

Call your doctor.

YES

Call your doctor.

If your infant is affected, is she also feeding poorly, and is she drowsy and unresponsive?

YES → Call your doctor.

Call your doctor.

YES

If your child is affected, does she have abdominal pain, vomiting with diarrhea, or 15 to 20 stools in 24 hours?

NO

If your child is affected, does she have: mucus in stools, bloody or black stools, sunken eyes, dry skin, drowsiness, or inability to urinate?

YES → Call your doctor.

NO

Try a self-care measure. Call your nurse information service or doctor if the diarrhea lasts more than 3 days after self-care.

NO ← Have you had diarrhea for more than a week or have you started taking a new medication?

YES

Call your nurse information service or doctor.

sure to take in enough fluids to replace what you're losing. If dehydration is a problem, *see* page 195.

- When you feel like you can tolerate solid foods, start with the BRAT diet: bananas, rice, applesauce, and dry toast.
- Cut out caffeine; it stimulates the intestine and can worsen your diarrhea. Dairy products, alcohol, and highly seasoned foods should also be avoided during diarrhea and for the first few days after it stops.
- If you suspect that lactose intolerance is causing your diarrhea, try lactose-free dairy products (available in most supermarkets), or buy a lactase-replacement product (available at most drugstores).

- Use over-the-counter antidiarrheals for very frequent bowel movements, but only if you do not have a fever over 101°F, severe abdominal pain, or blood in your stool.

Prevention

- To prevent food-associated gastrointestinal infection, follow the rules of safe food handling (*see* page 149).

DIZZINESS

The Problem

You have a sensation of being off-balance, whirling, or falling. The room may seem to be spinning around you.

Causes of Dizziness

Vertigo. You get dizzy when you lean forward or backward, move your head, look up or down, turn your head quickly, roll over in bed, or after vigorous exercise. It only lasts a few seconds. You may be middle-aged. Most of the time there's no apparent reason for it, though sometimes vertigo follows head trauma or occurs along with a stroke (*see* page 258). If it happens when you jump up suddenly, the blood has probably pooled in your lower legs, temporarily depriving your brain. This is usually harmless, unless it happens frequently and is associated with other symptoms.

Labyrinthitis. You have intense vertigo with nausea and perhaps vomiting. Your eyes move jerkily, and you may have ringing in your ears. It came on abruptly and has lasted for several hours or even days. The balance mechanism in the vestibular system and the semicircular canals of your inner ear have been disturbed, possibly by a viral inflammation.

Other Causes

Alcohol or drug use
Medication side effect
Hyperventilation (*see* page 48)
Migraine (*see* page 112)
Heat exhaustion
Epilepsy
Ménière's disease (*see* page 76)
Multiple sclerosis
Hypoglycemia
Anemia (*see* page 92)
Transient ischemic attack
  (*see* page 56)
Stroke (*see* page 258)
Cardiac *arrhythmia*
Brain *tumor*
Tumor

Self-Care Measures

- Move slowly, sit very still, and look straight ahead for a few minutes, or lie down until the dizziness goes away. For vertigo, repetitive head turning may improve symptoms by "fatiguing" the inner-ear vestibular system.

Prevention

- Avoid stress and tension; try relaxation techniques. If you are hyperventilating, try breathing into a paper bag (*see* page 48).
- Don't sit up or stand up suddenly. Don't jump out of bed, especially if you are middle-aged or older.

Treating Your Child

- Have your child lie down with legs propped up above head level.

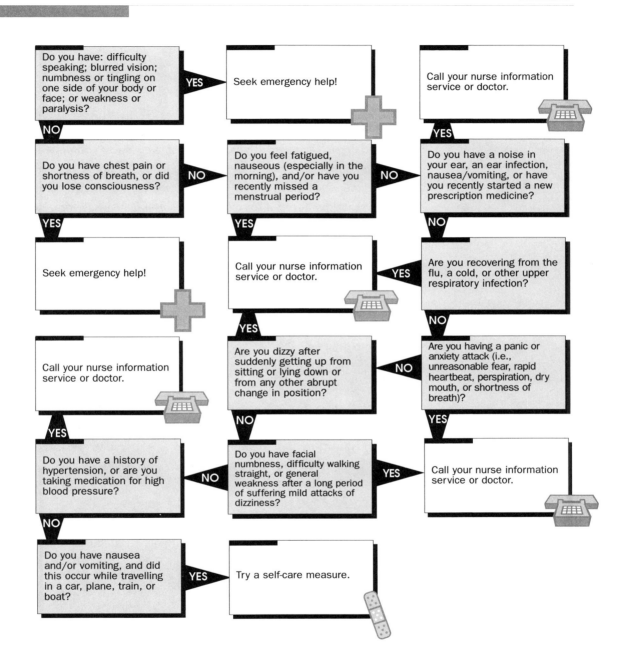

Do you have: difficulty speaking; blurred vision; numbness or tingling on one side of your body or face; or weakness or paralysis? **YES** → Seek emergency help!

NO ↓

Do you have chest pain or shortness of breath, or did you lose consciousness? **NO** → Do you feel fatigued, nauseous (especially in the morning), and/or have you recently missed a menstrual period? **NO** → Do you have a noise in your ear, an ear infection, nausea/vomiting, or have you recently started a new prescription medicine?

Call your nurse information service or doctor. **YES** ↑

YES ↓ (chest pain)

Seek emergency help!

YES ↓ (fatigued)

Call your nurse information service or doctor. **YES** → Are you recovering from the flu, a cold, or other upper respiratory infection?

NO ↓ (menstrual)

NO ↓ (recovering)

Call your nurse information service or doctor.

YES ↓ (dizzy)

Are you dizzy after suddenly getting up from sitting or lying down or from any other abrupt change in position? **NO** → Are you having a panic or anxiety attack (i.e., unreasonable fear, rapid heartbeat, perspiration, dry mouth, or shortness of breath)?

NO ↓ (dizzy)

YES ↓ (panic)

Do you have a history of hypertension, or are you taking medication for high blood pressure? **NO** → Do you have facial numbness, difficulty walking straight, or general weakness after a long period of suffering mild attacks of dizziness? **YES** → Call your nurse information service or doctor.

YES ↑ (hypertension)

NO ↓ (hypertension)

Do you have nausea and/or vomiting, and did this occur while travelling in a car, plane, train, or boat? **YES** → Try a self-care measure.

- Cool down with slow walking or other methods after strenuous exercise.
- Ask your nurse information service or doctor about special exercises to reduce the dizziness caused by head movement.

DROWSINESS

The Problem

You feel sleepy. You may not be getting enough sleep, or your sleep is not restful.

Other Causes

Insomnia (*see* page 130)
Common cold (*see* page 176)
Infection
Alcohol use
Caffeine withdrawal
Medication side effect
Narcolepsy
Encephalitis
Meningitis (*see* page 152)
Depression (*see* page 238)

Causes of Drowsiness

Inadequate sleep. The most common cause of drowsiness is simply not getting enough sleep. Most people underestimate the amount of sleep they need, and when they're very busy, they think that sufficient sleep is optional, rather than crucial for effective functioning. Most people need 7 to 8 hours of uninterrupted sleep each night; receiving less than that will likely lead to a drowsy feeling throughout the day.

Irregular sleep pattern. Sleeping at constantly changing or irregular times is another common cause of drowsiness. You may be working the late shift, or you're not going to bed and waking up at the same time every day. You may have disturbed the natural sleep/wake cycle.

Sleep apnea. Millions of people are believed to suffer from this sleep disorder, in which closures in the upper airway cause breathing to stop periodically. It is especially common in people who snore and are overweight. Usually, the brain, sensing that the body is not getting enough oxygen, will trigger a gasping reflex that partially awakens the person and restarts normal breathing. However, the result is that sleep is constantly interrupted and is not restful, leading to daytime drowsiness.

Self-Care Measures

- Get at least 7 hours of uninterrupted sleep in a 24-hour period. Sleeping isn't only something to do when you get a chance; it's essential to good health. Standardize your sleep patterns; try to go to bed and get up at the same time every day.

Treating Your Child

- See *Self-Care Measures* and *Prevention* listed here.

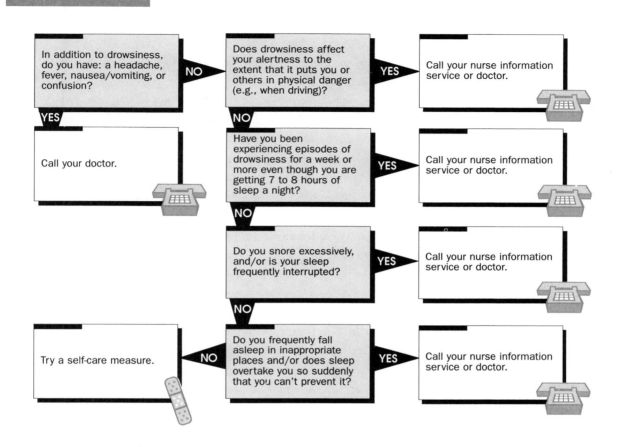

In addition to drowsiness, do you have: a headache, fever, nausea/vomiting, or confusion?

NO → Does drowsiness affect your alertness to the extent that it puts you or others in physical danger (e.g., when driving)?

YES → Call your nurse information service or doctor.

YES ↓

Call your doctor.

NO ↓ Have you been experiencing episodes of drowsiness for a week or more even though you are getting 7 to 8 hours of sleep a night?

YES → Call your nurse information service or doctor.

NO ↓ Do you snore excessively, and/or is your sleep frequently interrupted?

YES → Call your nurse information service or doctor.

NO ↓

Try a self-care measure. ← **NO** — Do you frequently fall asleep in inappropriate places and/or does sleep overtake you so suddenly that you can't prevent it?

YES → Call your nurse information service or doctor.

- If your schedule allows, try taking a nap in the middle of the afternoon. A 45-minute nap helps many people feel more alert (although some do find that it has the opposite effect). Don't do this if you have trouble sleeping at night.
- Drink caffeinated coffee, tea, or soft drinks, but don't overdo it; the equivalent of 1 or 2 cups of coffee in the morning and a cup in the afternoon is enough.
- Exercise. You're most likely to feel drowsy during periods when you're not physically active. Taking a walk, preferably in the sun, at the first sign of drowsiness may help.

Prevention

- Get at least 7 hours of uninterrupted sleep in every 24-hour period.
- Exercise.
- Limit your intake of coffee, tea, soft drinks, and other caffeinated products such as chocolate and some over-the-counter cold medications.

EAR, OBJECT IN

The Problem

You have a foreign object lodged in your ear. You may also have ear pain and hearing loss.

Important Information About Objects in the Ear

A variety of objects can end up in ears, especially children's ears; marbles, tiny toys, bits of paper, cotton swabs, jewelry, seeds, and earplugs are a few possibilities. It is also not unusual for insects to fly into human ears. The ear's structure prevents most objects from penetrating into the middle and inner ear, but it is possible for an object to scratch or perforate the eardrum. Perforation may be especially likely during attempts to remove objects. Therefore, if you or your child has an object lodged in the ear, follow the self-care measures below carefully.

Self-Care Measures

- If there is a foreign object lodged in your ear, follow these steps:
  - Cotton swabs are meant for cleaning the outside of the ears only. Don't use cotton swabs or any other tools to try to remove the object from the ear canal by probing at it; this increases the risk of pushing the object further into the ear.
  - Work with gravity's pull by tilting your head to the affected side. Gently shake your head in the direction of the ground to try to dislodge the object. (Do not strike your head.)
  - If this is ineffective, tilt the head in the other direction and make one attempt to remove the object with tweezers if the object is visible in the outer ear. (Further probing may cause injury.) If this doesn't work, call your nurse information service or doctor.

Treating Your Child
- See *Self-Care Measures* and *Prevention* listed here.

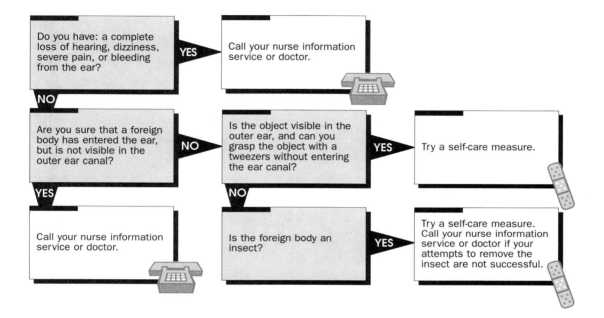

- If the foreign object is an insect, you can attempt to remove it by following these steps (Note: Do not use this technique unless you are certain that the object in the ear is an insect. Another foreign object might expand as a result of absorption of the liquid and become more difficult to remove):
  - Lie down on your side with the affected ear up.
  - Fill the ear canal, drop by drop, with oil (you can use mineral oil, baby oil, cooking oil, or olive oil) at room temperature. Gently pull the earlobe upward and backward to open the canal.
  - The insect will drown and float to the top. Blot it away with a tissue. Then lie on the opposite side to drain the remaining oil.

Prevention

- Never insert small objects into your ear.

EAR, RINGING IN

The Problem

You hear a buzzing, ringing, or hissing noise in your ear (tinnitus).

Causes of Ringing in the Ear

Other Causes

Hearing loss (*see* page 114)
Salicylate medication
Infection
Nerve damage (*see* page 114)
Perforated eardrum
Insect in the ear
Quinine
Arteriosclerosis
Brain *tumor*
Auditory nerve *tumor*

Barotrauma. Your earache began after you took an airplane trip or went deep-sea diving, especially if you started out with a cold or stuffy nose. You may also be experiencing dizziness, ringing in your ears, and a feeling that your ears are plugged or that you are talking in an echo chamber. Symptoms of barotrauma result from changes in air-pressure balance between the middle and outer ears, and they usually clear up on their own. If they do not go away after several days of decongestant therapy, however, treatment with antibiotics may be necessary.

Ménière's disease. You have tinnitus, vertigo (dizziness), fluctuating hearing loss, and pressure in your ear. This condition usually affects one ear, then both, apparently due to an increase of fluid in the labyrinth, that part of the inner ear most involved in balance.

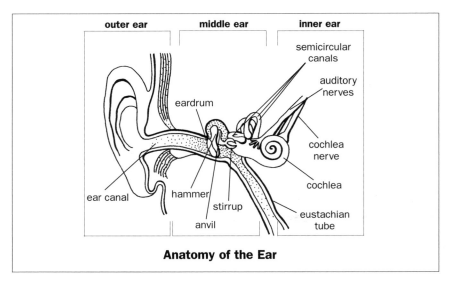

Anatomy of the Ear

Treating Your Child

- See *Self-Care Measures* and *Prevention* listed here.

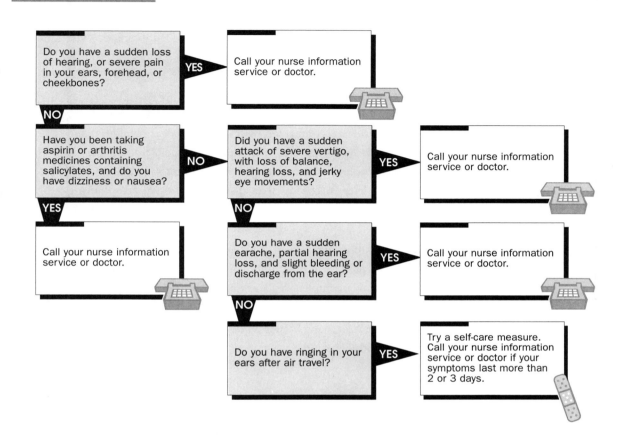

Do you have a sudden loss of hearing, or severe pain in your ears, forehead, or cheekbones?

YES → Call your nurse information service or doctor.

NO ↓

Have you been taking aspirin or arthritis medicines containing salicylates, and do you have dizziness or nausea?

NO → Did you have a sudden attack of severe vertigo, with loss of balance, hearing loss, and jerky eye movements?

YES → Call your nurse information service or doctor.

YES ↓

Call your nurse information service or doctor.

NO ↓

Do you have a sudden earache, partial hearing loss, and slight bleeding or discharge from the ear?

YES → Call your nurse information service or doctor.

NO ↓

Do you have ringing in your ears after air travel?

YES → Try a self-care measure. Call your nurse information service or doctor if your symptoms last more than 2 or 3 days.

Self-Care Measures

- For minor symptoms, try relaxation or biofeedback techniques and/or a "white noise" tape.
- For mild symptoms after air travel: Take a decongestant 3 to 4 times a day and blow gently through your nose while holding your nostrils closed.

Prevention

- Avoid air travel when you have a cold. Chew gum or suck on hard candy, especially during takeoff and landing.
- Wear earplugs when exposed to loud noises.
- Take aspirin (*see* page 27), caffeine, and alcohol in moderation, and don't use products containing nicotine.

EARACHE

The Problem

You have pain in one or both ears that is dull and throbbing or sharp and stabbing, and may range from mild to severe.

Causes of Earache

Other Causes

Otitis media
Barotrauma (*see* page 76)
Sinusitis (*see* page 256)
Trauma
Temporomandibular joint (TMJ) syndrome (*see* page 200)
Foreign body (*see* page 74)
Tonsillitis (*see* page 103)
Pharyngitis (*see* page 196)
Eustachian tube dysfunction
Bullous myringitis
Neuralgia
Tooth decay (*see* page 200)
Thyroiditis
Mastoiditis
Cyst

Infection. You have severe ear pain that may worsen when you pull on your earlobe and is accompanied by fever (especially in children) and possibly a sticky yellow, green, or bloody discharge. Although ear infections can occur in adults, they are most common in infants and children, who frequently show their discomfort through irritability. Ear infections need to be treated with antibiotics to kill the bacteria that cause them.

Cerumen (wax blockage). Everyone's ear canals make some wax; it is the body's way of protecting the canals. There can, however, be excessive wax buildup, causing a complete blockage and painful pressure on the very sensitive lining tissue. This must usually be removed by a doctor.

Swimmer's ear. Your earache started after swimming. Swimmer's ear can be relieved by drying up the water that has entered your ear.

Self-Care Measures

There are several steps you can take to relieve an earache. Remember,

Treating Your Child

- Don't give aspirin to anyone under 19 years of age! It may cause a rare but serious problem called Reye's syndrome. Instead, use ibuprofen or acetaminophen (*see* page 27) for fever or pain.
- Ear infections are very common in babies and young children and often very painful. They are usually a complication of an upper-respiratory infection. Since they can't express their discomfort in words, suspect an ear infection in any infant or young child who is constantly touching or tugging at one or both ears, has a fever, cries constantly despite being comforted, is particularly irritable when lying down, is not eating normally, or is unresponsive to loud noises or to the sound of your voice. But remember, children normally play with parts of their bodies, including their ears, and cry when they are left alone or feel bored. So, unless a child with a cold seems unreasonably uncomfortable, she probably does not have an ear infection.
- Hold babies with their heads elevated while breast- or bottle-feeding.

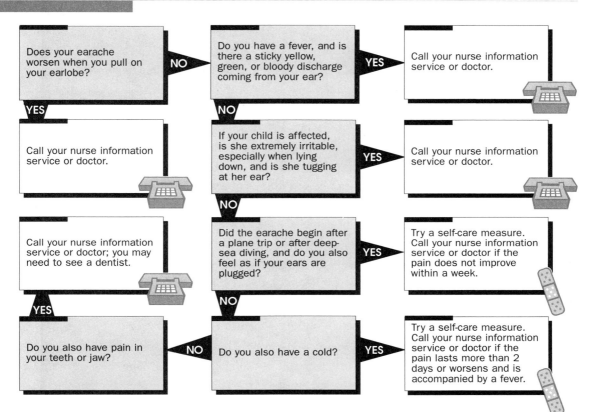

Does your earache worsen when you pull on your earlobe?

NO → Do you have a fever, and is there a sticky yellow, green, or bloody discharge coming from your ear?

YES → Call your nurse information service or doctor.

YES → Call your nurse information service or doctor.

NO → If your child is affected, is she extremely irritable, especially when lying down, and is she tugging at her ear?

YES → Call your nurse information service or doctor.

Call your nurse information service or doctor; you may need to see a dentist.

NO → Did the earache begin after a plane trip or after deep-sea diving, and do you also feel as if your ears are plugged?

YES → Try a self-care measure. Call your nurse information service or doctor if the pain does not improve within a week.

YES ← Do you also have pain in your teeth or jaw?

NO ← Do you also have a cold?

YES → Try a self-care measure. Call your nurse information service or doctor if the pain lasts more than 2 days or worsens and is accompanied by a fever.

however, that if your pain is caused by an infection, you will need an antibiotic prescription.

- To relieve pain, place a warm, wrung-out washcloth or a heating pad set on "low" next to your ear. Prop your head up when you sleep.
- Take an over-the-counter pain reliever, such as acetaminophen, aspirin, ibuprofen, or naproxen sodium (*see* page 27).
- Take an over-the-counter decongestant to dry up fluid in your ear.
- To dry up the water that causes swimmer's ear, try holding a hair dryer, set on "low," 10 to 12 inches from your ear, and aim the warm air into your ear canal. You can also try putting 1 to 2 drops of alcohol into your ear, which may help the water evaporate.

Prevention

- Shake your head to expel trapped water after swimming or showering, and use a hair dryer to dry out the ear canal. If you experience recurrent bouts of swimmer's ear, use alcohol and vinegar mix or an over-the-counter ear drop each time your ear canal gets wet. Also, don't remove ear wax before swimming; it coats the ear canal and protects it from moisture.
- Avoid air travel when you have a cold; or yawn, chew gum, or suck on hard candy during takeoffs and landings.
- If you tend to have excessive wax buildup, use an over-the-counter ear drop and ear irrigation kit every month or so after your doctor has completely removed all wax.
- Never insert small objects into your ear.

ELBOW PAIN

The Problem

You have pain in your elbow and perhaps swelling, tenderness, redness, or bruising.

Causes of Elbow Pain

Bursitis. You have swelling around the elbow; it's painful, especially when you press on it. You may have a fever. Your doctor may want to drain the fluid to be sure there's no infection and then will probably suggest a compression wrap, an anti-inflammatory medication such as aspirin or ibuprofen (see page 27), and avoidance of direct pressure.

Fracture/dislocation. You have fallen, or your elbow has been injured. It's swollen, bruised, or bleeding; looks twisted or deformed; and is painful, tender, hard to move, and stiff within a half hour after the injury. It may be *dislocated*, broken, or you may have chipped a bone or torn soft tissue around the elbow.

Compression injury. You have pain in your elbow and numbness and tingling in your fourth and fifth fingers. You've been repeatedly leaning your elbow on a hard surface, such as a desk, or the handlebars of a bicycle. You may have damaged your ulnar nerve, which passes under your elbow at a spot commonly referred to as the "funny bone." Try not to lean on your elbow, and use a protective pad when you do.

Tennis elbow. You have pain in the outer part of your elbow and upper forearm after repeatedly rolling or twisting the forearm, wrist, and hand (e.g., playing tennis or using a screwdriver or wrench). Try self-care and prevention measures.

Treating Your Child

- A young child who is pulled by the arm may dislocate his elbow. He will avoid using it and keep his arm flexed. A simple maneuver performed by your doctor will correct the problem.
- Most elbow injuries or sprains in children are easily cared for with ice and perhaps an elastic bandage or sling to rest the arm. If the pain lasts or is worse the following day, if the elbow is red and/or hot, or if your child has a temperature over 100°F, call your nurse information service or doctor.

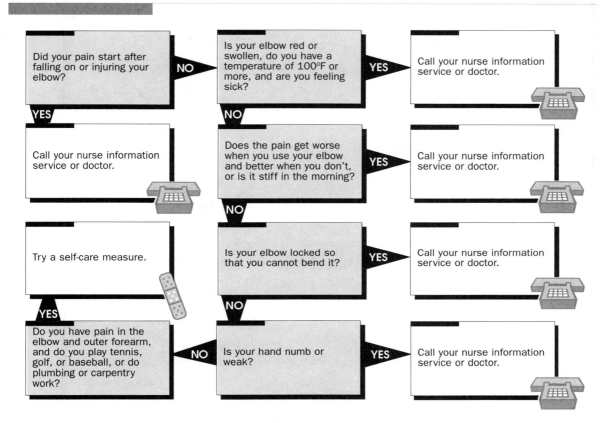

Did your pain start after falling on or injuring your elbow?

NO → Is your elbow red or swollen, do you have a temperature of 100°F or more, and are you feeling sick?

YES → Call your nurse information service or doctor.

YES → Call your nurse information service or doctor.

NO → Does the pain get worse when you use your elbow and better when you don't, or is it stiff in the morning?

YES → Call your nurse information service or doctor.

Try a self-care measure.

NO → Is your elbow locked so that you cannot bend it?

YES → Call your nurse information service or doctor.

YES → Do you have pain in the elbow and outer forearm, and do you play tennis, golf, or baseball, or do plumbing or carpentry work?

NO → Is your hand numb or weak?

YES → Call your nurse information service or doctor.

Self-Care Measures

- For the first 48 hours: Apply ice packs (20 minutes on, 20 minutes off). Rest your elbow, using a sling if needed. Avoid stress or strain on the joint. Try an over-the-counter anti-inflammatory pain reliever such as ibuprofen (*see* page 28).

- After 48 hours: Begin carefully moving your elbow through its range of motion every hour or so. Ask your nurse information service or doctor about elbow exercises.

Prevention

- Ask your nurse information service or doctor about exercises that will strengthen your forearm and shoulder.

- Use the proper equipment, posture, and movement for repetitive-motion activities (e.g., typing, using a screwdriver, playing golf or tennis, or pitching a baseball).

- For tennis elbow: Ask an instructor to correct your backhand; reduce your hours of play; warm up before playing; apply ice after a game; and use a tennis-elbow strap. Try ibuprofen (*see* page 28) an hour before and 6 hours after playing.

EYE DISCHARGE

The Problem

Your eyes are producing a clear or yellowish discharge, and they are also swollen, itchy, and red. They may also be stuck closed and crusty when you wake up.

Other Causes

Conjunctivitis (*see* page 84)
Blepharitis (*see* page 84)
Corneal ulcer or infection (*see* page 88)
Contact lens problem
Foreign object (*see* page 86)
Smog or other airborne eye irritant

Causes of Eye Discharge

Allergic reaction. You have been exposed to some kind of airborne irritant to which you are allergic, and now your eyes are teary, red, swollen, and itchy. Allergens such as pollen, dust, mold spores, animal dander (i.e., tiny scales from hair, feathers, or skin), chlorinated water, cosmetics, or even contact lens solutions often cause allergic reactions that affect your eyes. The most effective way to relieve these reactions is to avoid the offending allergen, but if you can't do that, self-care measures can help.

Bell's palsy. You have drooping muscles on one side of your face, along with weakness on that side, drooling, and possible pain in the ear, changes in taste, and increased sensitivity to noise. Bell's palsy results from inflammation of the facial nerve, but it is not certain what causes it.

Stye. You have a small, red, painful bump on your upper or lower eyelid. You also feel as if there is something in your eye, and are tearing excessively. Styes are caused by a bacterial infection of an eyelash follicle. Squeezing the bump may spread the infection and cause other styes to develop.

Treating Your Child

- Conjunctivitis is very common in children, because of their frequent exposure to other children with similar problems and because they tend to rub their eyes with dirty hands. Remind your child to keep his hands clean and not to rub his eyes if he tends to get recurrent conjunctivitis.

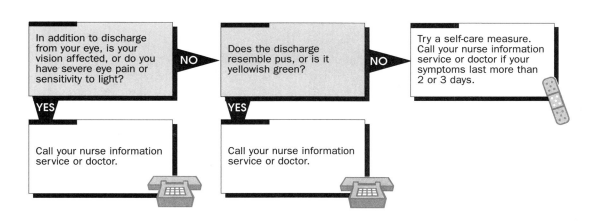

Self-Care Measures

- For conjunctivitis:
  - If your eyes are crusted shut when you wake up, loosen the crusts with a warm, wrung-out washcloth. Don't use this washcloth again until it is laundered.
  - Wash your eyelids with a cotton ball dipped in a solution of a half-teaspoon of salt dissolved in a teaspoon of warm water.
  - Apply a washcloth soaked in warm water to your closed eyes for 5 minutes, 3 or 4 times a day.
  - To relieve itching and irritation, try over-the-counter eyedrops.
  - Throw out any eye makeup that you were using when the infection started, and don't wear eye makeup while you have an eye infection.
  - Don't wear a patch over your eye; covering the eye may allow an infection to spread.
  - Contact lenses should not be worn while you have an infection.

- For styes:
  - To relieve eye irritation resulting from a stye, apply a warm compress (run a clean cloth under hot water) to the area for a 10-minute period, 3 or 4 times a day.
  - Never squeeze a stye; the swelling will go down on its own.
- If allergens are the cause, use antihistamines and eyedrops for relief.

Prevention

- When you have an eye infection, wash your hands often and don't share washcloths and towels. This will help to prevent the infection from spreading to others.
- Don't ever share eye makeup, eyedrops, or contact lens supplies with others.
- Carefully clean contact lenses and replace old lenses.

EYE, ITCHY/RED

The Problem

Your eye is itchy and/or red.

Causes of Eye Itch/Redness

Other Causes

Allergy
Foreign body (*see* page 86)

Bacterial conjunctivitis ("pinkeye"). Your eyes are itchy, red, and swollen, with a thick, whitish or yellowish discharge. Your eyes are also stuck shut when you wake up. Conjunctivitis, or "pinkeye," is an inflammation of the membrane that covers the white of the eye and the inner surface of the eyelids; this particular type of conjunctivitis is caused by a bacterial infection. It is potentially serious because it can cause ulceration of the *cornea*. It must be treated with antibiotic eyedrops. Untreated pinkeye can permanently impair vision. It's highly contagious and is quite commonly caused by sharing eye makeup.

Viral conjunctivitis ("pinkeye"). Your eyes are itchy, red and swollen, and they are producing a clear, watery discharge. "Pinkeye" that is caused by a virus usually has symptoms that are less severe and bothersome than those of bacterial conjunctivitis. Viral conjunctivitis may be a complication of a cold (*see* page 176) or *influenza*, and it can take several days to clear up. Because the cause is viral, antibiotics won't help.

Keratitis. Your eyes are inflamed and painful, but you have no other symptoms. You've been wearing your hard contact lenses longer than recommended, or you've been overexposed to sunlight. Your corneas may be injured.

Blepharitis. Your eyes are red and itchy. The eyelid edges are inflamed and scaly. This condition often accompanies dandruff. If self-care measures don't work or your symptoms are severe, call your nurse information service or doctor. You may require an ointment and warm salt water rinses for the eye.

Treating Your Child

- See *Self-Care Measures* and *Prevention* listed here.

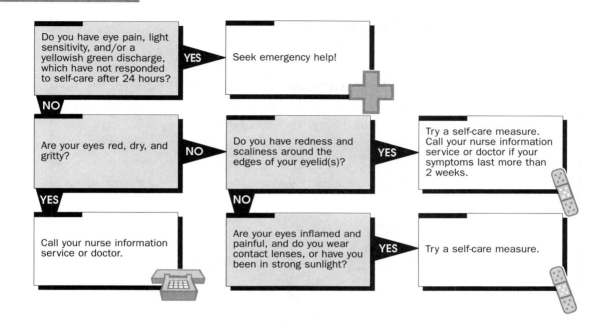

Dry eye. Your eyes are red and dry, and you have few or no tears. The white of your eye is red and swollen, and your eye feels hot and gritty. Dry eye sometimes accompanies rheumatoid arthritis (*see* page 224). It occurs more often in women than men and is a frequent complaint during menopause.

Self-Care Measures

- If conjunctivitis is the cause, *see* page 83.
- For keratitis, take an over-the-counter pain remedy, don't wear contact lenses, and wear an eye patch until you can see your doctor.
- For blepharitis, wash away the scales twice a day with warm water or baby shampoo.
- For dry eye, you can relieve the discomfort with over-the-counter artificial tears.
- If you have a painless red patch on the white of your eye that appears suddenly, leave it alone. It is usually harmless and will clear up on its own.
- To relieve redness, use a clean cloth to apply a cool compress.

Prevention

- To avoid the spread of pinkeye, wash your hands often, don't share washcloths or towels, and launder these frequently. Never share eye makeup.
- For keratitis, follow strict instructions for contact lens cleaning and use; do not exceed recommended time limits for wearing contact lenses.
- Wear UV-protective lenses in strong sunlight.
- Eliminate all possible allergens, including perfumed tissues, cosmetics, and detergents.

EYE, OBJECT IN

The Problem
You have a foreign object in your eye.

Important Information About Objects in the Eye
Most specks that enter the eye are harmless and can be taken care of by blinking or tearing. You should never try to remove an object if it is embedded in your *cornea*, if your eye is obviously injured, if you suddenly have severe pain or trouble seeing, or if you develop a fever. You may have an injury that poses a serious threat to your sight.

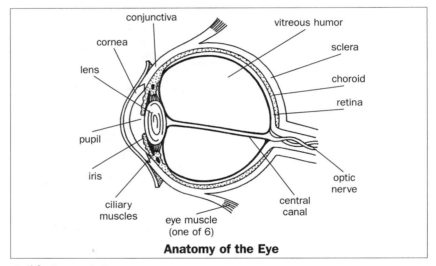

Anatomy of the Eye

Self-Care Measures
When attempting to remove an object from your eye, do not rub your eye or try to remove an object that is stuck or embedded. Instead, cover both eyes with a sterile or clean compress and call your nurse information service or doctor or have someone make the call for you. It is important to cover both eyes because if the unaffected eye is open the pupils in both eyes will change in reaction to light exposure, potentially

Treating Your Child
- See *Self-Care Measures* and *Prevention* listed here.

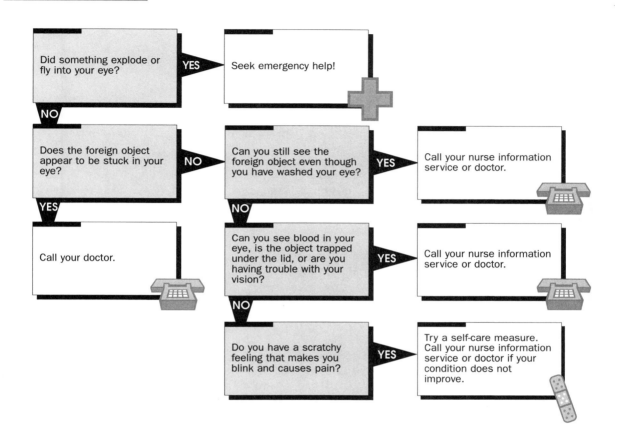

Did something explode or fly into your eye? — **YES** → Seek emergency help!

NO ↓

Does the foreign object appear to be stuck in your eye? — **NO** → Can you still see the foreign object even though you have washed your eye? — **YES** → Call your nurse information service or doctor.

YES ↓

Call your doctor.

NO ↓

Can you see blood in your eye, is the object trapped under the lid, or are you having trouble with your vision? — **YES** → Call your nurse information service or doctor.

NO ↓

Do you have a scratchy feeling that makes you blink and causes pain? — **YES** → Try a self-care measure. Call your nurse information service or doctor if your condition does not improve.

worsening your eye pain. If you can't close your eye, cover it with a small paper cup.

- To remove an object that is not stuck in your eye but is on the surface or under your eyelid:
  - Wash your hands; then gently pull down your lower eyelid. If the object is there, remove it with the tip of a moistened cotton swab or the corner of a clean cloth.
  - If the object is not visible, grasp the eyelashes of the upper eyelid and pull out and down until the upper lid overlaps the lower. Wait a moment until your tears wash the object out.

  - If the object is still there, wash the eye using eye irrigating solution or open your eye under running water.
  - For lingering pain or discomfort after an object is removed, call your nurse information service or doctor.

Prevention

- Always wear protective eye gear when doing carpentry, metalwork, heavy yard maintenance, or any activity involving loose dirt, wood splinters, sawdust, metal, glass, or any other particles.

EYE PAIN

The Problem

Your eye hurts, feels scratchy, throbs, or is sharply painful.

Causes of Eye Pain

Other Causes

Foreign object (*see* page 86)
Glaucoma (*see* page 230)
Sinusitis (*see* page 256)
Conjunctivitis (*see* page 84)
Dry eye (*see* page 84)
Meningitis (*see* page 150)
Blepharitis (*see* page 84)
Burn from welding or
   ultraviolet light
Iritis
Uveitis

Eyestrain. Your eyes feel tired and you may have a headache. If your vision is blurred at close distance or your ablility to focus on objects at close range has gotten worse, you may need eyeglasses or contact lenses.

Injury. You have sudden pain in your eye, decreased vision, or redness after being struck. Many eye injuries can be avoided by taking preventative measures while playing sports or participating in other potentially hazardous activities.

Corneal ulcer or infection. You have severe eye pain, blurred vision, excess tears, light sensitivity, and difficulty keeping your eyelids open without severe pain.

Self-Care Measures

- Rest your eyes.
- Wear sunglasses to protect your eyes from bright light or ultraviolet rays.
- Use cool or warm compresses (whichever gives the most relief) several times a day for an hour.
- Sleep with your head elevated for a few days.
- Try artificial tears to relieve dryness or irritation.

Treating Your Child
- See *Self-Care Measures* and *Prevention* listed here.

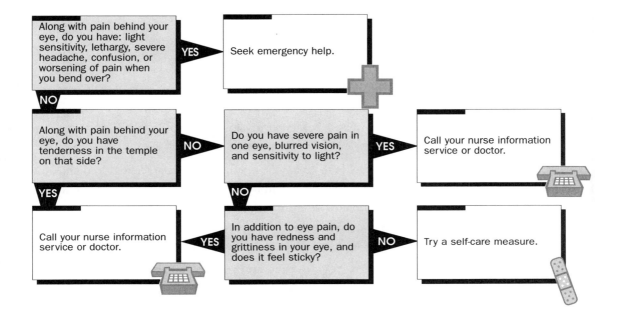

Prevention

- Wear protective eye gear while playing sports, doing carpentry, or working in construction.
- Keep your contact lenses clean, don't leave them in too long, and remove them as soon as you feel eye pain.
- Be careful when using anything near your eyes. Makeup brushes, fingernails, and sprays can scratch or irritate the *cornea*.
- Avoid tanning salons; if you do use them, wear appropriate eye protection.

FAINTNESS

The Problem
You briefly lose consciousness.

Causes of Faintness

Other Causes

Hypotension (low blood pressure)
Pregnancy
Heat exposure
Dehydration
Head injury (*see* page 110)
Transient ischemic attack
  (*see* page 56)
Bleeding *ulcer*
Epilepsy
Fear or an unpleasant sight
Arrhythmia
Medication side effect

Postural hypotension. You feel dizzy or faint when you sit up or stand suddenly. This is due to a sudden drop in blood pressure. It has many causes and is especially common in the elderly, following a meal. If it happens often, remember to get up slowly, and discuss it with your doctor during your next appointment.

Anemia. You feel faint or have fainted. You've been feeling tired and weak and looking pale; and you may have shortness of breath; rapid heartbeat when you exert yourself; loss of weight (*see* page 214) and appetite (*see* page 34); a sore, red tongue; bleeding gums (*see* page 104); or nosebleeds (*see* page 155).

Low blood sugar. You are faint, and you feel hungry, anxious, and irritable. You are perspiring and trembling, and you may also have palpitations, confusion, and loss of coordination. Prompt intake of sugar or carbohydrates may relieve the fainting, but you should consult your nurse information service or doctor.

Self-Care Measures
- Make sure the person who has fainted is lying down, breathing, and has a pulse. Raise the legs above the head, loosen clothing, and make the person comfortable.
- Don't sit up or stand immediately on regaining consciousness. Weakness after fainting is common.

Treating Your Child
- See *Self-Care Measures* and *Prevention* listed here.

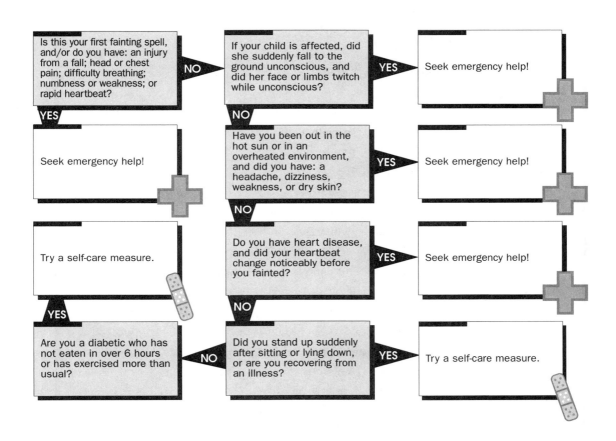

Is this your first fainting spell, and/or do you have: an injury from a fall; head or chest pain; difficulty breathing; numbness or weakness; or rapid heartbeat?

NO → If your child is affected, did she suddenly fall to the ground unconscious, and did her face or limbs twitch while unconscious?

YES → Seek emergency help!

YES → Seek emergency help!

NO → Have you been out in the hot sun or in an overheated environment, and did you have: a headache, dizziness, weakness, or dry skin?

YES → Seek emergency help!

Try a self-care measure.

NO → Do you have heart disease, and did your heartbeat change noticeably before you fainted?

YES → Seek emergency help!

YES → Are you a diabetic who has not eaten in over 6 hours or has exercised more than usual?

NO → Did you stand up suddenly after sitting or lying down, or are you recovering from an illness?

YES → Try a self-care measure.

- If you are diabetic and haven't eaten for 6 hours, try dried fruit or orange juice. Ask your doctor for other snack ideas.
- If you are pregnant, avoid standing for prolonged periods; move around to stimulate circulation.
- If you have low blood sugar, carry glucose tablets, sugar, or candy to eat when you feel faint, or drink fruit juice.

- Drink plenty of liquids, especially in hot weather. *Dehydration* can trigger or aggravate faintness. Avoid alcohol.

Prevention
- Don't sit up or stand suddenly. Stay hydrated by drinking plenty of fluids. Eat three meals a day.

FATIGUE

The Problem

You are tired or lack energy.

Causes of Fatigue

Other Causes

Boredom or stress
Depression (*see* page 238)
Medication side effect
Caffeine withdrawal
Drug use
Intestinal parasite
Heart disease (*see* page 236)
Liver disease
Kidney disease
Cancer
Chronic infection
Sickle cell anemia

Lifestyle. You stay up very late several nights a week and sleep late several mornings. You eat an unbalanced diet heavy on junk food, get very little exercise, diet on and off, smoke, drink excessively, and work too hard. You need a change in lifestyle to combat your fatigue.

Infection. You have profound fatigue, low-grade fever, and swollen glands in your neck. You could have mononucleosis, viral *hepatitis,* or—if your fatigue has lasted for at least 6 months—*chronic fatigue syndrome.* If you also have aching joints and a headache and have been in an area infested with ticks, you could have Lyme disease.

Anemia. You feel faint and a little breathless, you look pale, and you may have palpitations. Anemia may be the cause, especially if you are a woman who has heavy menstrual periods, if you eat a diet low in iron, or if you have suffered blood loss. Self-care measures can help.

Hypothyroidism. You are a middle-aged woman who is feeling tired all the time and having difficulty keeping warm. Your hair may be thinning a little, and your skin is dry. An underactive thyroid gland could be the problem and can be treated.

Self-Care Measures

- Regulate your sleep; try to sleep the same 7 to 8 hours every night.
- Start a program of moderate, regular exercise; reduce your activity if you've been working out excessively.
- If anemia is the cause, you should eat plenty of whole-grain bread, dried fruit, and leafy green vegetables (*see* figure). Iron supplements may also help. Ask your doctor whether you need other treatment.

Treating Your Child

- See *Self-Care Measures* and *Prevention* listed here.

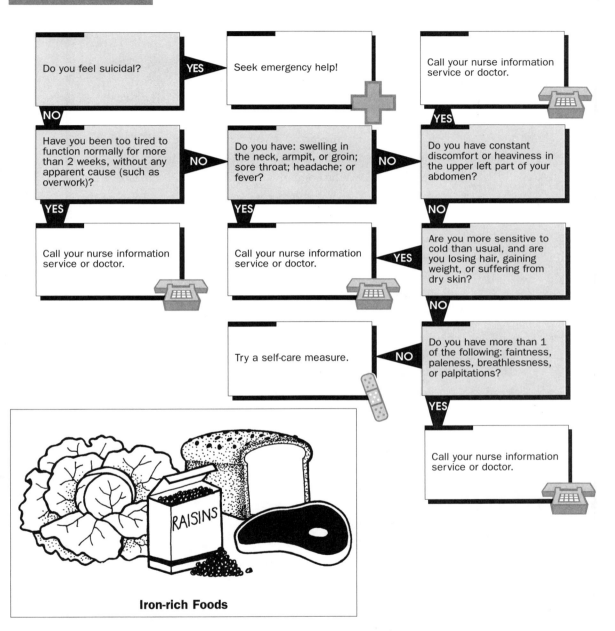

Do you feel suicidal?

YES → Seek emergency help!

NO ↓

Have you been too tired to function normally for more than 2 weeks, without any apparent cause (such as overwork)?

NO → Do you have: swelling in the neck, armpit, or groin; sore throat; headache; or fever?

YES ↓ Call your nurse information service or doctor.

YES → Call your nurse information service or doctor.

Call your nurse information service or doctor.

YES ↑

Do you have constant discomfort or heaviness in the upper left part of your abdomen?

NO ↓

Are you more sensitive to cold than usual, and are you losing hair, gaining weight, or suffering from dry skin?

YES → Call your nurse information service or doctor.

NO ↓

Try a self-care measure.

NO ← Do you have more than 1 of the following: faintness, paleness, breathlessness, or palpitations?

YES ↓

Call your nurse information service or doctor.

Iron-rich Foods

- Eat a healthy, balanced diet, and drink plenty of water.
- Learn some relaxation and stress-relieving techniques.

Prevention

- Regulate your sleep, eat a balanced diet, and stay hydrated by drinking plenty of fluids. Avoid stimulant medications, caffeine, and alcohol.

FEVER

The Problem

Your temperature is over 100°F (or 101°F in a child over 1 year). You feel hot and sweaty or hot and chilled. Untreated temperatures are generally at their highest from 4 p.m. to 10 p.m.

Other Causes

Sore throat
Pneumonia
Bronchitis
Sinusitis (*see* page 256)
Hepatitis
Diarrhea (*see* page 68)
Cholecystitis
Allergy
Sunstroke and heat exhaustion (*see* page 194)
Mononucleosis (*see* page 102)
Meningitis (*see* page 150)
Appendicitis

Causes of Fever

Viral and bacterial infections. If your fever is below 103°F and you have a mild sore throat, aches and pains, headache, runny nose, or sneezing, you probably have the common cold (*see* page 176) or *influenza*. However, if you become short of breath, even while at rest, or if you cough up discolored sputum, it could be *pneumonia* or *bronchitis*.

Kidney, urinary tract, or female reproductive infection. Your fever (usually over 102°F) is sudden, with shaking chills and burning, frequent urination. There may be blood or yellow vaginal discharge. Your lower back hurts, sometimes severely, and you might feel nauseated. Fever right after childbirth or pain in your lower abdomen, with smelly or heavy vaginal discharge, signals serious infections in women.

Self-Care Measures

- Take an over-the-counter medication containing aspirin, acetaminophen, or ibuprofen if not contraindicated (*see* page 27).
- Sponge with tepid water. Bath water that is about 70°F lowers fever and is more comfortable than very cold water. Dress in light, loose clothes, and use light bedcovers.

Treating Your Child

- Don't give aspirin to anyone under 19 years of age! It may cause a rare but serious problem called Reye's sydrome. Instead, use ibuprofen or acetaminophen (*see* page 27) for fever or pain.
- Fever seizures (i.e., high temperature "fits") are fairly common among children, usually last only a minute (rarely more than 5) and are basically harmless. However, seizures lasting longer can be dangerous, so in addition to calling your nurse information service or doctor, follow these steps immediately:

- Reduce the fever with sponging or bathing in tepid water. Check temperature every half hour until it drops below 102°F; then stop sponging. Have her lie down.
- Make sure the child can breathe. Clear food or vomit from the mouth, and gently move the head till the neck is arched, or stretched out, and the head is turned to the side.
- For the next few days, watch carefully for fever or signs of another convulsion.

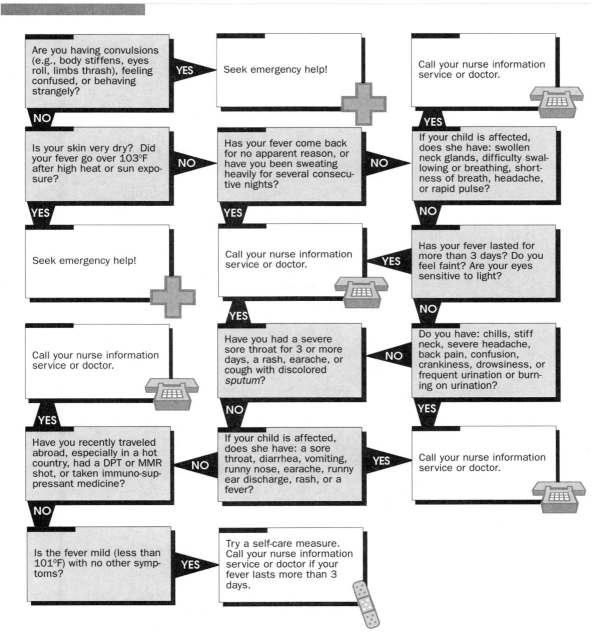

Are you having convulsions (e.g., body stiffens, eyes roll, limbs thrash), feeling confused, or behaving strangely?

YES → Seek emergency help!

NO ↓

Is your skin very dry? Did your fever go over 103°F after high heat or sun exposure?

NO → Has your fever come back for no apparent reason, or have you been sweating heavily for several consecutive nights?

YES ↓

Seek emergency help!

Call your nurse information service or doctor.

YES ↑ (to top right)

If your child is affected, does she have: swollen neck glands, difficulty swallowing or breathing, shortness of breath, headache, or rapid pulse?

Call your nurse information service or doctor.

YES ↑

Call your nurse information service or doctor.

YES → Has your fever lasted for more than 3 days? Do you feel faint? Are your eyes sensitive to light?

NO ↓

YES ↓

Have you had a severe sore throat for 3 or more days, a rash, earache, or cough with discolored *sputum*?

NO ← Do you have: chills, stiff neck, severe headache, back pain, confusion, crankiness, drowsiness, or frequent urination or burning on urination?

YES ↑

Have you recently traveled abroad, especially in a hot country, had a DPT or MMR shot, or taken immuno-suppressant medicine?

NO ← If your child is affected, does she have: a sore throat, diarrhea, vomiting, runny nose, earache, runny ear discharge, rash, or a fever?

YES → Call your nurse information service or doctor.

NO ↓

Is the fever mild (less than 101°F) with no other symptoms?

YES → Try a self-care measure. Call your nurse information service or doctor if your fever lasts more than 3 days.

- Drink plenty of fluids, including water, juices, teas, broths, and sports drinks, to replace lost nutrients and prevent dehydration. Eat if you're hungry, but don't force it.

Prevention

- Take appropriate steps to protect yourself against some of the causes of fever, such as overexposure to heat and sun, or close contact with people suffering from high fever.

FINGER PAIN/INJURY

The Problem

You have pain in your finger.

Causes of Finger Pain and Injury

Other Causes

Animal bite (*see* page 39)
Osteoarthritis (*see* page 224)
Frostbite
Rheumatoid arthritis
  (*see* page 224)
Raynaud's disease
  (*see* page 156)
Carpal tunnel syndrome
  (*see* page 216)

Injury. The most common injury involves crushing your finger, either in a door or with a hammer. Some such injuries will heal by themselves, others are more serious.

Tenosynovitis (repetitive strain disorder). You have trouble straightening your finger; then suddenly it snaps straight (called "trigger finger" when it happens in your index finger). The synovium, or membrane, covering the tendon has become inflamed and narrowed so it stops movement briefly until the tendon can overcome the obstruction and suddenly jerk free. It may make a crackling sound. The condition is sometimes caused by infection, but more often by repetitive movement, such as typing or working on an assembly line.

Severed tendon. You have cut your finger severely across an area where the tendons run lengthwise from the wrist to the fingertips, and you can't move one or more fingers.

Paronychia. You have red, swollen skin alongside your nail. You may have gotten a superficial yeast, herpes, or staphylococcal infection after pulling off a hangnail (a bit of skin hanging loose at the side or root of a fingernail) or pushing back your cuticle (the layer of skin attached to the base of the nail that helps protect the growth of new nail cells).

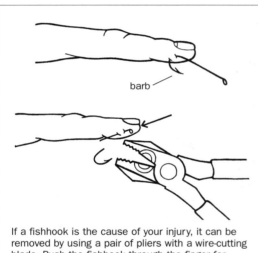

barb

If a fishhook is the cause of your injury, it can be removed by using a pair of pliers with a wire-cutting blade. Push the fishhook through the finger far enough to see the pointed barb, cut the hook right below the barb, and pull the hook out backward.

Self-Care Measures

- If paronychia is the cause, try hot soaks twice daily (5 to 10 minutes),

Treating Your Child

- See *Self-Care Measures* and *Prevention* listed here.

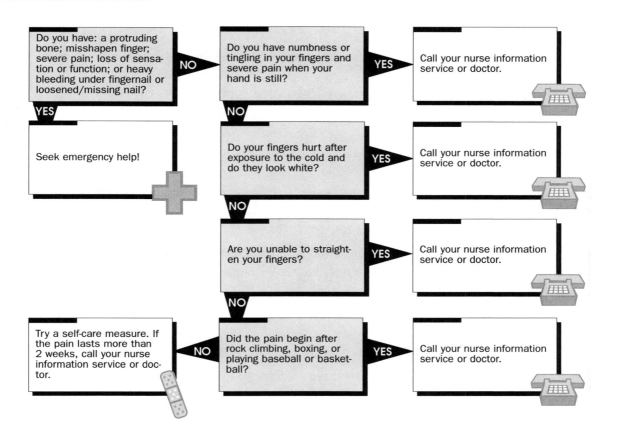

Do you have: a protruding bone; misshapen finger; severe pain; loss of sensation or function; or heavy bleeding under fingernail or loosened/missing nail?

NO → Do you have numbness or tingling in your fingers and severe pain when your hand is still? **YES** → Call your nurse information service or doctor.

YES → Seek emergency help!

NO → Do your fingers hurt after exposure to the cold and do they look white? **YES** → Call your nurse information service or doctor.

NO → Are you unable to straighten your fingers? **YES** → Call your nurse information service or doctor.

NO → Try a self-care measure. If the pain lasts more than 2 weeks, call your nurse information service or doctor. ← **NO** ← Did the pain begin after rock climbing, boxing, or playing baseball or basketball? **YES** → Call your nurse information service or doctor.

to reduce inflammation, followed by an antibacterial medication or 1% gentian violet for fungal infections.

- If your fingers are crushed, try the RICE remedy: rest, ice, compression, and elevation. Rest your fingers for a day or so; you can resume activity gradually as you find that you're able to tolerate it. During the rest period, apply ice several times a day, 10 minutes on and 10 minutes off. Compress your fingers by wrapping them snugly, but not tightly, with an elastic bandage. And finally, keep your fingers elevated to drain fluids away from the joint.

- Stretch knobby joints gently a couple of times a day by straightening your hands out on a tabletop, then making a fist and cocking your wrist back to increase stretch. Use the other hand to very gently bend and straighten out each finger.
- Take prescribed anti-inflammatory medicine, but avoid strong pain relievers; these may mask severe pain that could indicate a more serious problem.
- Use a moist heating pad or a warm, wet towel to wrap a painful joint.

Prevention

- Avoid repetitive strain by varying activities or taking frequent breaks.

FOOT PAIN/ITCH

The Problem

You have pain, itching, swelling, or irritation in one or both of your feet.

Causes of Foot Pain and Itch

Other Causes

Corn or callus (*see* page 60)
Bunion
Blister (*see* page 42)
Stress *fracture*
Plantar fasciitis
Contact dermatitis (*see* page 178)
Gout (*see* page 108)
Hammertoe (*see* page 198)
Mallet toe (*see* page 198)
Arthritis (*see* page 224)
Flat feet
Neuropathy
Diabetes (*see* page 240)

Athlete's foot. Your foot or feet sting, itch, and burn, especially between and underneath your third, fourth, and fifth toes. Your skin is also reddened, cracked, scaly, and peeling. Athlete's foot, a fungal infection, is mildly contagious and is transmitted by contact in public showers, locker rooms, and swimming areas, or by sharing towels or footwear with someone who has the fungal infection. It is not serious, but it can be very uncomfortable.

Morton's neuroma. You have burning pain and cramping above your third and fourth toes. Morton's neuroma usually affects women who wear tight shoes.

Calcaneal spur. You have an overgrowth of the heel bone that places pressure on the other structures in the heel, that may result in irritation. It may be associated with *plantar fasciitis*.

Plantar warts. You have small lumps with one or more little black dots in the middle, on the bottom of your foot or feet. They are contagious and may cause pain.

Self-Care Measures

- If you have athlete's foot, good foot hygiene is crucial. Wash your feet up to 4 times a day with warm water and soap, and dry them thoroughly using a hair dryer set on its coolest setting. Put on clean cotton socks. Allow your feet to air out as often as possible, and

Treating Your Child

- Young children might not be able to tell you when their shoes are too tight, so have your child's foot measured at a shoe store at least 3 times a year. Make sure your child's shoes fit comfortably.

- Children may get an itchy, red rash on the bottom of both feet if they are allergic to a material in the shoes. This is common with tennis shoes. Have your child wear a different shoe type and go barefoot inside.

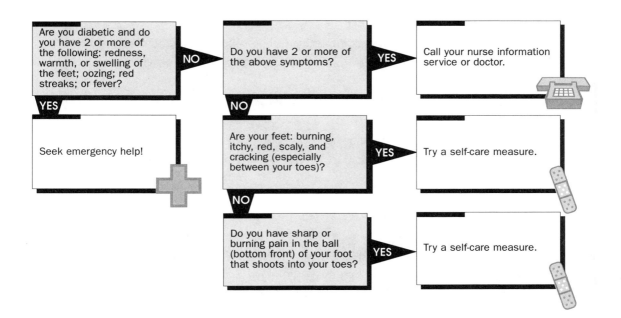

Are you diabetic and do you have 2 or more of the following: redness, warmth, or swelling of the feet; oozing; red streaks; or fever?

NO → Do you have 2 or more of the above symptoms?

YES → Call your nurse information service or doctor.

YES ↓

Seek emergency help!

NO ↓

Are your feet: burning, itchy, red, scaly, and cracking (especially between your toes)?

YES → Try a self-care measure.

NO ↓

Do you have sharp or burning pain in the ball (bottom front) of your foot that shoots into your toes?

YES → Try a self-care measure.

---

wear only shoes that let your feet breathe. (Avoid plastic shoes or shoes that are lined with plastic.) Use an over-the-counter antifungal lotion or cream. Use antifungal powder during the day when you must wear shoes and socks, and antifungal creams at night.

- If a corn or callus is the cause, *see* page 60.
- If you have Morton's neuroma, wearing wider and flatter shoes and simply massaging your foot usually provide relief.
- If plantar warts are the cause, *see* page 212.
- Use orthotic-type arch supports, heel cushions, and foot exercises along with an ice massage after being on feet.

Prevention

- Many foot problems are caused by wearing shoes that are too tight, and they can be prevented by wearing shoes that fit comfortably. If you're not certain that your shoes are the right size for you, have your feet professionally measured at a shoe store. If your feet tend to swell as the day goes on have your foot measured in the morning, and elevate your feet throughout the day whenever possible, especially during hot weather. Limit your intake of salt. Be sure to have your feet remeasured after having a baby; you're likely to find that they've grown by at least a half size!
- To prevent athlete's foot, keep your feet as clean and dry as possible. If you're treating a plantar wart or a case of athlete's foot, wear slippers, shower sandals, or socks around the house and locker room to prevent transmission of the infection to others.

99

GAS/FLATULENCE

The Problem

You have an uncomfortable feeling of fullness in your abdomen, your stomach rumbles, and you belch or frequently expel gas rectally.

Other Causes

Indigestion
Swallowing air
Nutrient malabsorption
   (*see* page 214)
Hiatal hernia (*see* page 118)
Lactose intolerance (*see* page 68)
Irritable bowel syndrome
   (*see* page 186)
Inflammation of the colon
Giardia
Slow stomach emptying

Causes of Gas and Flatulence

Gas-producing food. Your problem usually occurs after consuming high-fiber foods such as beans, bran, or fibrous vegetables, or beverages containing yeast (e.g., beer) or carbonation. Self-care measures should relieve the problem.

Self-Care Measures

- Eat slowly, and reduce your intake of gas-producing foods, including apples, beans, bran, broccoli, cabbage, cauliflower, nuts, onions, peaches, pears, popcorn, prunes, and soybeans.
- If lactose intolerance is the cause, *see* page 69.
- Do not chew gum or drink through a straw.

Treating Your Child

- See *Self-Care Measures* and *Prevention* listed here.

Prevention

- If gas and flatulence are a significant problem for you, alter your diet to reduce your intake of gas-producing foods, beer, dairy products, and carbonated drinks.

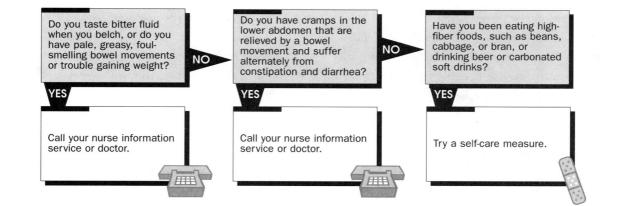

Do you taste bitter fluid when you belch, or do you have pale, greasy, foul-smelling bowel movements or trouble gaining weight? **NO** → Do you have cramps in the lower abdomen that are relieved by a bowel movement and suffer alternately from constipation and diarrhea? **NO** → Have you been eating high-fiber foods, such as beans, cabbage, or bran, or drinking beer or carbonated soft drinks?

YES → Call your nurse information service or doctor.

YES → Call your nurse information service or doctor.

YES → Try a self-care measure.

GENITAL SORE

The Problem

You have a bump, blister, wart, or rash on your penis or vagina or in the genital area.

Other Causes

Herpes (*see* page 42)
Genital warts (*see* page 212)
Penile cancer (*see* page 158)
Scabies (*see* page 132)
Vaginal *cancer*
Infection
Trauma
Friction

Causes of Genital Sores

Syphilis. You have a hard, red, painless, ulcerating sore on your genitals called a chancre (pronounced "shanker"). Avoid sexual contact until you've completed treatment. Any sexual partners in recent months should be informed.

Self-Care Measures

- If herpes is the cause, *see* page 43.

Prevention

- Avoid sexual contact with anyone who has sores on the genitals, anus, or tongue, or who complains of genital tingling or irritation.
- To prevent infecting others, always use a latex condom for all sexual contact.

Treating Your Child

- See *Self-Care Measures* and *Prevention* listed here.

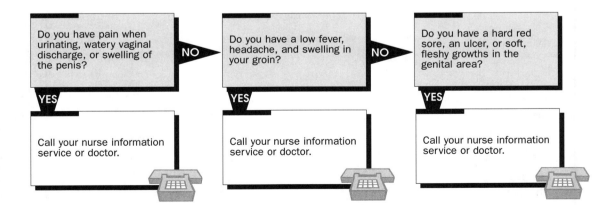

Do you have pain when urinating, watery vaginal discharge, or swelling of the penis?

NO →

Do you have a low fever, headache, and swelling in your groin?

NO →

Do you have a hard red sore, an ulcer, or soft, fleshy growths in the genital area?

YES ↓

Call your nurse information service or doctor.

YES ↓

Call your nurse information service or doctor.

YES ↓

Call your nurse information service or doctor.

GLANDS, SWOLLEN

The Problem

You have a lumpy swelling just below, in front of, or behind your ears, down both sides or on the back of your neck, or in your armpit or groin (*see* figure).

Other Causes

Strep throat (*see* page 196)
Skin irritation
Chronic fatigue syndrome
Diphtheria
Abscessed tooth (*see* page 200)
HIV infection (*see* page 242)
Leukemia
Hodgkin's lymphoma
Breast *cancer*
Head *cancer*
Neck *cancer*

Causes of Swollen Glands

Infection. Your glands are swollen in two or more places (i.e., your neck, armpit, or groin). You may have a fever and a general feeling of being sick. Many viruses can cause swollen glands. Scalp infections may cause swelling in the back of the neck; foot infections, including ordinary athlete's foot, can cause swollen glands in the groin. Certain sexually transmitted diseases can also cause groin swelling.

Mononucleosis. Your neck, groin, and armpit glands are swollen, and you have a high fever, severe sore throat, and trouble swallowing.

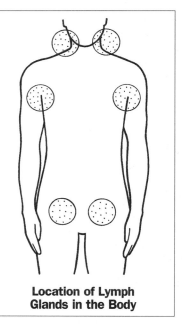

Location of Lymph Glands in the Body

Mumps. You have swelling between the angle of your jaw and your ears. You may have low fever, earache, headache, and fatigue. You have been exposed to someone with mumps and have not been immunized.

German measles. You or your child have swollen glands in the back of the neck and, within a couple of days, a pink rash on your body. This is

Treating Your Child

- Don't give aspirin to anyone under 19 years of age! It may cause a rare but serious problem called Reye's syndrome. Instead, use ibuprofen or acetaminophen (*see* page 27) for fever or pain.
- Warm compresses and plenty of cold liquids to drink are comforting.
- Don't force a child to eat solid foods if it hurts him to swallow.

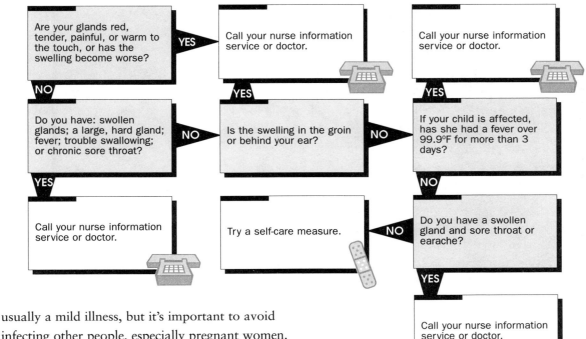

usually a mild illness, but it's important to avoid infecting other people, especially pregnant women.

Tonsillitis. Your child complains of having a sore throat and doesn't want to eat anything solid. The glands are swollen on the sides of her neck. You can make her more comfortable with self-care. If she doesn't get better in 48 hours, if her symptoms get worse, or if she has any new symptoms, call your nurse information service or doctor.

Self-Care Measures

- If you are very uncomfortable, apply a warm compress (a washcloth soaked in warm water, for example) as often as needed, and take aspirin, acetaminophen, or ibuprofen (*see* page 27). Tenderness or soreness usually goes away in a couple of days; swelling may take several weeks to go down. If it doesn't, if it gets worse, or if other glands become swollen, call your nurse information service or doctor.

- If you have mononucleosis, avoid sports or activities in which your *spleen* (located in your upper left side, below your ribs) might be hit; it may be enlarged and could rupture.

Prevention

- Exposure to viruses and bacteria is so common that prevention is nearly impossible. However, mumps and measles are preventable by immunization. Make sure you and your children are immunized.

GUMS, BLEEDING

The Problem

Your gums bleed easily.

Causes of Bleeding Gums

Other Causes

Blood clotting disorder

Gingivitis. Your gums are red, soft, shiny, and swollen. They bleed easily, even from gentle brushing. Gingivitis can be prevented by proper dental hygiene. However, once started, it can lead to serious gum and jawbone disease if not treated.

Periodontal disease. You have untreated gingivitis. Your gums bleed easily. Plaque—a sticky deposit of debris and bacteria—collects in pockets between your swollen gums and your teeth. You may have an unpleasant taste in your mouth and bad breath. The gum pulls back from the base of your teeth, exposing areas that are sensitive to hot, cold, or sweet foods or drinks. Sometimes an abscess forms deep inside one of your gum-line pockets. The bone around the base of your teeth is being destroyed, and one or more of your teeth may be loose. This is a serious condition.

Anemia or *leukemia*. If your gums bleed easily, and you also have nosebleeds, fatigue and weakness, shortness of breath, and a tendency to bruise easily, you may have a severe anemia. If you have those symptoms plus bone pain—especially in your legs—abdominal pain and swelling, nausea, fever, night sweats, and decreased appetite or weight loss, you may have a type of leukemia.

Vincent's infection ("trench mouth"). You have red, swollen, painful, bleeding gums with a grayish film. It hurts to speak or swallow, and you have bad breath and a bad taste in your mouth. You salivate excessively. This is a noncontagious infection associated with poor dental hygiene, physical or emotional stress, poor nutrition, and heavy smoking. It must be treated, and the irritating causes (e.g., smoking or spicy foods) must be eliminated.

Treating Your Child

- See *Self-Care Measures* and *Prevention* listed here.

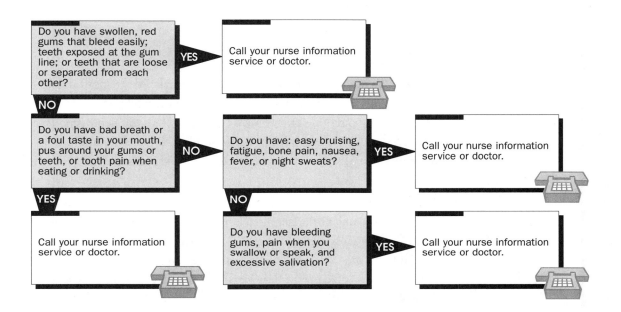

Self-Care Measures

- Brush your teeth thoroughly with a fluoride toothpaste at least twice a day and after each meal if possible. Use dental floss at least once a day. Use a disclosing tablet occasionally to see if you're cleaning your teeth well enough.
- Watch your diet! Avoid foods with large amounts of refined sugar, especially foods that stick to your teeth. Eat foods with roughage (e.g., green vegetables and apples). Finish your meals with a little cheese to counteract acidity.
- Get plenty of vitamins A and C every day. Cantaloupe, broccoli, spinach, liver, fortified dairy products, oranges, grapefruit, tomatoes, potatoes, and green peppers are good sources.
- Have your teeth professionally cleaned twice a year.

Prevention

- Brush your teeth twice a day, use dental floss at least once a day, avoid foods containing large amounts of refined sugar, get plenty of vitamins C and A every day, and visit your dentist at least twice a year.

HAIR LOSS

The Problem

Your hair is thinning or falling out at an abnormal rate.

Causes of Hair Loss

Other Causes

Aging
High fever (*see* page 94)
Medication side effect
Fungal infection
Damaging hair-care technique
Cancer chemotherapy
Malnutrition
Trichotilomania (constant pulling
   or tugging of the hair)

Alopecia areata. You've quickly lost all of the hair in one spot or several patches, but you have no infection or other illness, and your scalp is normal. This common condition may be due to tension, depression (*see* page 238), other emotional factors, or no identifiable cause at all. It often goes away, with new hair covering the bald spots in 6 to 9 months, with no treatment.

Male pattern baldness. Your hair has slowly thinned and begun to disappear, starting at the temples or front of your scalp and working back over the crown of the head. An inherited condition, it may be related to an increased sensitivity to androgen (i.e., "male" hormone) and is not reversible. You can wear a toupee or try hair-weaving or transplantation if your lack of hair concerns you.

Ringworm. You have bald patches on your scalp, scaly patches of skin, and itching. You may also have *pustules* and oozing. Remedies applied to the scalp won't get rid of the fungus in the hair shafts. You may need a prescription for an oral antifungal medication.

Hypothyroidism. Your hair is sparse, coarse, and dry, and you have unexplained fatigue (*see* page 92), weight gain (*see* page 213), muscle

Treating Your Child

- Infants often lose their fine baby hair, especially if they rub their heads against mattresses, chairs, or car seats. Stronger hair will eventually replace it.
- When children lose hair, it is often because of tight braids or ponytails, hair-pulling by friends and siblings or themselves. If a child persistently pulls his own hair, call your nurse information service or doctor.
- If ringworm is the cause, wash the child's hairbrush or comb often during treatment to prevent reinfection. Also wash caps, barrettes, and hair ties. Hair will grow back normally after treatment.

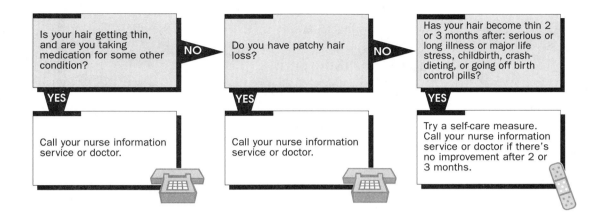

pain, cramps, intolerance for cold, constipation (*see* page 58), dry skin (*see* page 178), and heavier periods. You have an underactive thyroid gland and will need to take synthetic thyroid supplements.

Excess androgen in women. Your hair is becoming thin at the temples or at the crown of your head, while becoming thicker or more noticeable on your face. You may also have abnormally oily skin. Too much "male" hormone may be genetic or due to menopausal changes or medications, especially birth control pills or menopausal hormone-replacement therapy. This imbalance can usually be corrected. Rarely this may be caused by a *tumor* of the ovaries or adrenal glands that secretes androgen hormone.

Self-Care Measures

- Avoid very alkaline shampoos.
- Don't towel-dry too vigorously or use a hot hair dryer; let hair air-dry whenever possible.
- Comb; don't brush.

- Wigs, hair transplants, weaving, and topical *minoxidil* are options, but all are expensive and limited in their effect. Women respond better than men to minoxidil. Do not use minoxidil if you are under 18 or if you have heart problems. Do not use on babies and children, or if you are pregnant or nursing a baby.
- Don't regularly braid or ponytail your hair tightly, use a curling iron or hot curlers, or have your hair bleached, permed, or dyed.

Prevention

- Pay attention to good nutrition.
- Treat your hair gently.
- Avoid excessive professional hair modifications.
- Limit use of chlorinated pools.
- Avoid sharing combs and brushes, which can transmit infections.

HAND PAIN

The Problem

You have pain, swelling, and/or redness in your hand.

Causes of Hand Pain

Other Causes

Sprain or strain (*see* page 182)
Carpal tunnel syndrome
  (*see* page 156)
Arthritis (*see* page 224)
Cervical osteoarthritis
  (*see* page 156)
Spondylosis
Juvenile rheumatoid arthritis
Diabetes (*see* page 240)
Raynaud's disease (*see* page 156)

Tendinitis. Your fingers are painful and tender, with tenderness worsening at night. You also have trouble moving your fingers and you may have muscle *spasms* in your hand. Tendinitis is caused by sudden physical trauma (e.g., falling or lifting heavy objects), prolonged repetitive movement. It can affect any part of the body but most commonly affects the shoulders, elbows, wrists, ankles, and fingers.

Ganglia. You have a round swelling under the skin of your wrist or the back of your hand. It may be hard or rubbery but usually not painful or tender. You have a ganglion or ganglionic *cyst*, which is common and usually needs no treatment. If especially troublesome, it can be aspirated (i.e., emptied) with a needle in your doctor's office or removed surgically.

Infection. You have pain, swelling, redness, and warmth in your hand. You also have a fever and feel ill. This could be *osteomyelitis* (especially if there was any preceding trauma to the hand), *infectious arthritis*, soft tissue infection, or rheumatic fever (especially if you recently had a sore throat).

Gout. You have pain in the joint at the base of your big toe, foot, ankle, or knee, or in your hand or elbow, that has intensified to the point that no position provides relief. Gout is actually a type of arthritis (*see* page 224). It runs in families, and it results from a buildup of uric acid in the blood and around the joints. If your doctor diagnoses you with gout, you will probably receive antigout drugs and be advised to cut down on rich foods and alcohol.

Treating Your Child

- Children don't commonly have joint pain in their hands, unless they've been injured.

If your child has joint pain and fever, call your nurse information service or doctor.

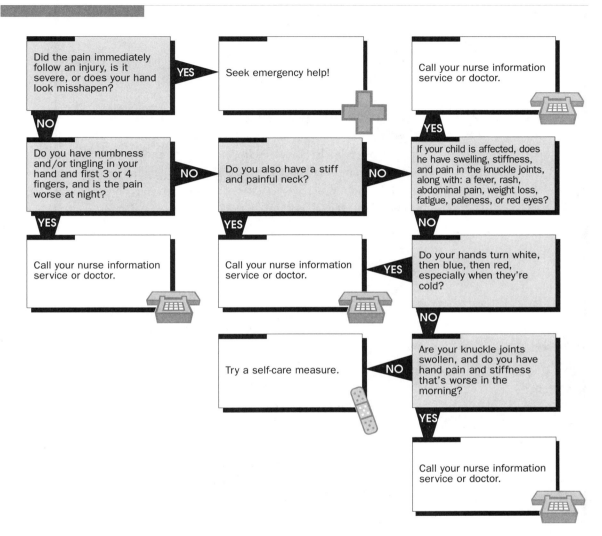

Self-Care Measures

- If tendinitis is the cause, try the RICE remedy (*see* page 182).

Prevention

- For sprains, strains, tendinitis, and carpal tunnel syndrome:
  - Avoid highly repetitive movement.
  - Take breaks.
  - Use appropriate arm and wrist supports while keyboarding.
  - Vary your activities.
- Exercise regularly at a level you are comfortable with, warming up and cooling down before and after your workout.
- Use the proper sports equipment (e.g., the right gloves, wrist guards, or protective gear, etc.).

HEAD INJURY

The Problem

You have sustained an injury to your head, with or without loss of consciousness or other visible signs.

Important Information About Head Injuries

The best approach to head injuries is to take precautions to prevent them in the first place by driving carefully and wearing protective headgear when appropriate. The most severe head injuries generally result from automobile and motorcycle accidents. The most serious consequences of a head injury are concussion, intracranial hematoma, and skull fracture.

Concussion. A hard blow to the head creates a sudden movement of the brain within the skull. A concussion usually involves a loss of consciousness, loss of memory, dizziness, and vomiting.

Intracranial hematoma. A blood vessel ruptures between the skull and the brain, and the blood that leaks out forms a hematoma (i.e., blood clot) that puts pressure on brain tissue. As the pressure increases, symptoms such as headache, nausea, vomiting, confusion, loss of strength or feeling, and changes in pupil size may occur (*see* figure).

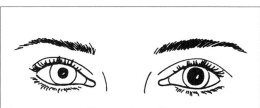

Unequal pupils

Skull fracture. This is a break in the bone that surrounds and protects the brain. It usually results from a head injury. Symptoms of skull fracture include bruising or discoloration behind the ear or around the eyes, blood or clear fluids leaking from the ears or nose, unequal size of pupils, or swelling or depression of the skull.

Self-Care Measures

- Patients who have sustained any sort of head injury will need to be

Treating Your Child

- Children frequently sustain minor head injuries. Watch for the symptoms listed in the flowchart. As long as the child remains conscious (even if initially stunned), is easily aroused from sleep (even if very drowsy), and has pupils that are the same size, the injury is probably minor. Call your nurse information service or doctor if you're concerned.

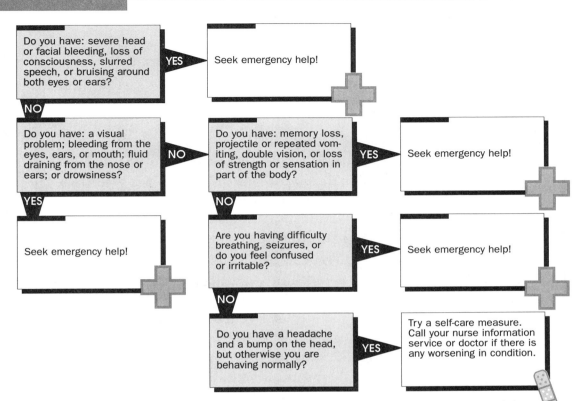

Do you have: severe head or facial bleeding, loss of consciousness, slurred speech, or bruising around both eyes or ears?

YES → Seek emergency help!

NO

Do you have: a visual problem; bleeding from the eyes, ears, or mouth; fluid draining from the nose or ears; or drowsiness?

NO → Do you have: memory loss, projectile or repeated vomiting, double vision, or loss of strength or sensation in part of the body?

YES → Seek emergency help!

YES → Seek emergency help!

NO

Are you having difficulty breathing, seizures, or do you feel confused or irritable?

YES → Seek emergency help!

NO

Do you have a headache and a bump on the head, but otherwise you are behaving normally?

YES → Try a self-care measure. Call your nurse information service or doctor if there is any worsening in condition.

watched carefully for the first 24 to 72 hours after the injury, since this is the period during which symptoms of serious problems occur. In most cases, however, this can be done as safely at home as it can in the hospital. Check the patient every 2 hours during the first 24 hours, every 4 hours during the second 24 hours, and every 8 hours during the third 24 hours. Look for the following, and call your nurse information service or doctor immediately if you note any of the symptoms listed in the flowchart above or:

– Noticeable restlessness.
– Pupils of unequal size or shape (*see* figure).
– Severe headache that continues for longer than 4 hours after the injury.

• You may be able to decrease swelling from a bump on the head by applying ice to the area. Remember, though, that the size of the bump is

not an indicator of the severity of the injury.

Prevention

• An alarming number of head injuries occur as a result of motorcycle accidents. It is crucial that riders wear helmets, whether or not state laws require them.

• Bicycle riders, skaters, and those involved in contact sports (especially football or boxing) should wear protective headgear at all times.

• Automobile drivers and passengers should wear seat belts and shoulder harnesses (*see* page 21). Young children should be placed in approved car seats. Never drive while under the influence of alcohol or mind-altering drugs.

• Avoid shaking an infant. Without direct injury to the head, an infant can sustain severe brain injury.

HEADACHE

The Problem

Your head hurts. The pain may be constricting and dull, throbbing or pounding, or sharp and stabbing. It may or may not be accompanied by other symptoms, such as nausea or dizziness.

Other Causes:

Fever (*see* page 94)
Sinusitis (*see* page 256)
Caffeine and alcohol withdrawal
Medication side effect
Hypertension (*see* page 244)
Abscessed tooth (*see* page 200)
Temporomandibular joint (TMJ) syndrome (*see* page 200)
Trauma
Cranial arteritis
Meningitis (*see* page 150)
Infection
Glaucoma (*see* page 230)
Stroke (*see* page 258)

Causes of Headache

Tension. You feel a dull, steady pressure in your head—it may feel like there is a tight elastic band around your head—and it worsens as the day goes on. Tension, or muscular, headaches occur when you strain the muscles of your head and neck, often without even realizing you have done it. These headaches are by far the most common.

Migraine. Your head throbs, especially on one side or behind your eyes, and this intense pain often starts in the morning. You may also feel nauseated and be extremely light- or noise-sensitive, and you may see flashing lights or spots before your eyes. Migraines are more common in women than in men, and they tend to run in families. They occur when the blood vessels in the scalp expand, and they may be triggered by certain factors, like stress, eating cheese or chocolate, drinking red wine, fasting, or exercising in bright, hot sunlight.

Treating Your Child

- Don't give aspirin to anyone under 19 years of age! It may cause a rare but serious problem called Reye's syndrome. Instead, use ibuprofen or acetaminophen (*see* page 27) for fever or pain.
- Headaches are unusual in children under the age of 3, except as a direct result of injury. In such a case, seek emergency help!
- Headaches in children over the age of 3 can be symptomatic of a number of problems, but they can also occur and disappear on their own. If your child has any of the following symptoms along with headache, call your nurse information service or doctor right away: drowsiness; stiff neck with increased pain when the head is bent forward; refusal to drink; fever over 100°F; vomiting without diarrhea; weakness; loss of coordination; or consistent, or early morning awakening from sleep due to headache.

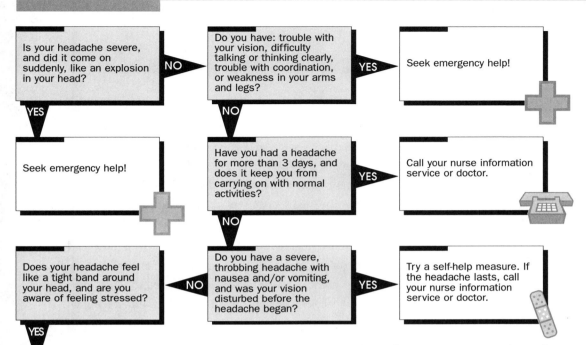

Is your headache severe, and did it come on suddenly, like an explosion in your head? — **NO** →

Do you have: trouble with your vision, difficulty talking or thinking clearly, trouble with coordination, or weakness in your arms and legs? — **YES** → Seek emergency help!

YES ↓

Seek emergency help!

NO ↓

Have you had a headache for more than 3 days, and does it keep you from carrying on with normal activities? — **YES** → Call your nurse information service or doctor.

NO ↓

Does your headache feel like a tight band around your head, and are you aware of feeling stressed? ← **NO** — Do you have a severe, throbbing headache with nausea and/or vomiting, and was your vision disturbed before the headache began? — **YES** → Try a self-help measure. If the headache lasts, call your nurse information service or doctor.

YES ↓

Try a self-care measure.

Self-Care Measures

• Take an over-the-counter pain reliever, such as aspirin, acetaminophen, or ibuprofen (*see* page 27), as soon as you feel a headache coming on. These medications can be very effective, especially when taken early; but if you find that you are using them several times a day or for extended periods of time, call your nurse information service or doctor.

• Tension headaches can often be relieved by massage (rub the base of your head with your thumbs, starting under your ears and working back and then up to your temples) or by applying heat to the back of your upper neck.

• If your headache is severe, it may be a migraine. Rest in a dark, quiet room with your eyes closed at the first sign of an attack. Put a cold washcloth or icepack over your eyes or icepack on your forehead. If these measures don't help, call your nurse information service or doctor. You may need prescription medication.

Prevention

• Keep track of when and where you get headaches so that you can avoid triggers.

• Eat regularly during the day, but be aware that there are certain foods and beverages that give some people headaches. Alcohol, bananas, caffeine, chocolate, food additives (e.g., monosodium glutamate), nitrates (found in hot dogs and other processed meats), hard or aged cheese, nuts, red wine, some artificial sweeteners (e.g., aspartame), and vinegar are examples.

• If you grind your teeth at night, buy a rubber bite-guard at a sporting-goods store and try wearing it while you sleep.

HEARING LOSS

The Problem

You have decreased ability or complete inability to hear some or all sounds in one or both ears.

Other Causes

Ménière's disease (*see* page 76)
Infection
Medication side effect
Otosclerosis
Ear injury
Head injury (*see* page 110)
Multiple sclerosis
Syphilis (*see* page 101)
Brain *tumor*
Auditory nerve *tumor*
Sensorineural loss

Possible Causes of Hearing Loss

Aging. You're probably over 60, and you've noticed that people seem to be mumbling a lot, you can't hear in church or in theaters, and your family keeps asking you to turn down the volume on the TV and radio. These are signs of age-related hearing loss, a condition called presbycusis.

Nerve damage. You are often exposed to loud noises or high-decibel sound, like that of jet engines, machinery, gunshots, or very loud music, and you notice that you can't hear as well as you used to. Such exposure can actually deaden the sensitive nerve endings that conduct sound.

Earwax blockage. Your hearing loss has come on gradually, and you feel as though your ears are blocked or filled with wax. Self-care measures will usually correct this problem.

Self-Care Measures

- If age-related hearing loss is the problem, ask people to speak clearly, distinctly, and in a normal tone. Call your nurse information service or doctor and ask whether a hearing aid would be helpful.

Treating Your Child

- Children can be born with a hearing deficit, or they can develop hearing loss as a result of frequent ear or upper respiratory tract infections. Consider the possibility of hearing loss if your infant doesn't seem to respond to environmental sounds, especially those that should be startling (e.g., a whistle or a loud clap).

- At about 4 months of age a baby begins to respond noticeably to sound. Consider the possibility of hearing loss if your child does not respond to your voice and is slow in learning how to speak (children usually learn to speak at around 1 year of age).

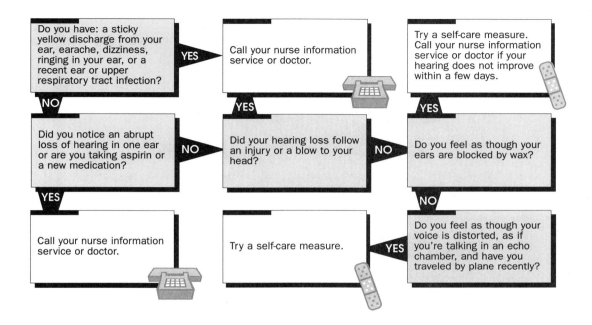

- To remove wax: Lying on your side, use a syringe without a needle or medicine dropper to carefully squeeze a few drops of lukewarm water into your ear. Let the water remain there for 10 to 15 minutes, and then shake it out. Repeat this procedure, but this time use a few drops of hydrogen peroxide, mineral oil, or an over-the-counter earwax remover. Let the excess fluid flow out of your ear. Then, after several minutes, repeat the procedure once more, this time with warm water. (Note: Do not use a cotton swab to remove earwax, and do not use the above procedure if your eardrum is injured or perforated.)

- Hearing may be impaired by colds, allergies, or recent plane trips. Using a decongestant (look for the ingredient pseudoephedrine) along with "popping" your ears several times a day will usually correct this. You can pop your ears by holding your nose, bearing down as if straining to have a bowel movement, and swallowing. If you have heart disease, diabetes, hyperthyroidism, or if you are pregnant or nursing a baby, you should call your nurse information service or doctor before using pseudoephedrine. Do not use monoamine oxidase inhibitors (MAOIs) or caffeine while taking pseudoephedrine.

Prevention

- Avoid exposure to high-decibel sound or, if frequent exposure is unavoidable, buy a pair of well-fitting earplugs. If you use portable headphones, keep the volume low.

- Don't put cotton swabs, fingers, bobby pins, or any small objects into your ear. Blow your nose gently; don't use too much force.

HEARTBEAT, RAPID

The Problem

Your heart is beating rapidly, and you're very aware of it. You may or may not be experiencing other symptoms as well.

Causes of Rapid Heartbeat

Other Causes

Anxiety or stress
Fever (*see* page 94)
Caffeine use
Cigarette smoking
Hyperthyroidism (*see* page 192)
Hypoglycemia
Anemia (*see* page 92)
Congestive heart failure
  (*see* page 234)
Diabetes mellitus (*see* page 240)
Blood loss
Dehydration
Alcohol withdrawal
Pulmonary embolus
Sickle cell anemia

Overexertion. You've just run up several flights of stairs, and now your heart is beating very fast. Physical exertion is a very common cause of rapid heartbeat. A heart rate as high as 160 beats per minute is not unusual with exercise and is generally not dangerous, as long as you are not experiencing other symptoms, like chest pain or faintness, and as long as your general health is good and you are less than 60 years old.

Medication side effect. You're taking an over-the-counter cold tablet, and you're having episodes of very rapid heartbeat; it may even feel as if your heart is beating out of your chest. Several over-the-counter and prescription medications can cause rapid heartbeat as a side effect. Examples include appetite suppressants, antihistamines, antidepressants, asthma relievers, and decongestants (e.g., pseudoephedrine and phenylpropanolamine hydrochloride, which are ingredients in many over-the-counter decongestants, are frequent offenders). If you are taking one of these medications and are experiencing episodes of rapid heartbeat, you may need to switch medications.

Heart disease. Your heart is beating rapidly, and you also have shortness of breath with minimal exertion. Heart disease (*see* page 236) is a possible cause of rapid heartbeat and it is almost always accompanied by other symptoms, such as breathlessness (*see* page 48), chest pain (*see* page 54), fainting (*see* page 90) or light-headedness, or fluid retention.

Treating Your Child
- See *Self-Care Measures* and *Prevention* listed here.

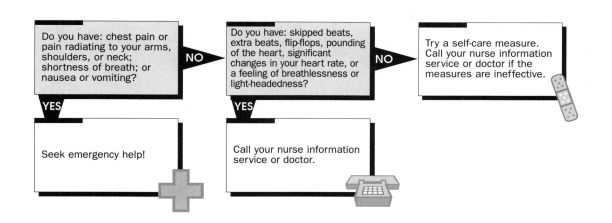

Do you have: chest pain or pain radiating to your arms, shoulders, or neck; shortness of breath; or nausea or vomiting?

NO

Do you have: skipped beats, extra beats, flip-flops, pounding of the heart, significant changes in your heart rate, or a feeling of breathlessness or light-headedness?

NO

Try a self-care measure. Call your nurse information service or doctor if the measures are ineffective.

YES

Seek emergency help!

YES

Call your nurse information service or doctor.

Self-Care Measures

Your normal heart rate should be 60 to 100 beats per minute. Most cases of rapid heartbeat are caused by anxiety, smoking, or taking in too much caffeine or alcohol. If the episodes pass quickly, and if you're not experiencing other symptoms at the same time, it's probably nothing to worry about. Try the following self-care measures.

- Cough a couple of times.
- Take a couple of swallows of ice-cold water.
- Hold your nose closed, and blow gently through your nostrils until your ears "pop."

- Relax and take deep breaths. If you feel dizzy, sit or lie down to avoid falling.
- Make a note of when your rapid heartbeat happens and what you are doing at the time. Also record any symptoms and how long they lasted. Count the number of beats per minute. Give this information to your doctor.

Prevention

- Do not smoke (*see* page 24).
- Watch your intake of alcohol, caffeinated coffee, tea, and cola.

HEARTBURN

The Problem

You have a burning pain just below your ribs or breastbone within an hour after a meal. You may feel stomach acid backing up into your throat, especially if you bend forward or lie down.

Other Causes

Peptic ulcer (*see* page 252)

Causes of Heartburn

Irritation. Irritation resulting from *stomach-acid reflux* can be caused by eating heavy meals; eating too fast; eating chocolate, garlic, onion, peppermint, tomato, or citrus fruit; lying down or smoking after a meal; drinking alcohol or coffee (including decaf); taking aspirin; wearing tight clothing; or being excessively overweight. Stress and emotional upset can also trigger heartburn.

Pregnancy. Hormonal changes, along with increased abdominal pressure, often produce heartburn.

Hiatal hernia. Part of the stomach may stick up through the diaphragm allowing stomach acid to squirt up because of a poorly functioning valve between the stomach and *esophagus*.

Esophageal ulcer. These are a result of chronic acid indigestion, which inflames the *esophagus* and causes erosion or narrowing.

Self-Care Measures

- To relieve pain, take a liquid nonprescription antacid (without calcium). If you have heart or kidney disease or high blood pressure (*see* page 244), call your nurse information service or doctor before taking an antacid.
- Drink skim milk or, if it's unavailable, water, to wash the acid down.

Prevention

The goal is to avoid anything that causes or encourages acid backup. If you have heartburn rather frequently, you may be able to identify the

Treating Your Child

- See *Self-Care Measures* and *Prevention* listed here.

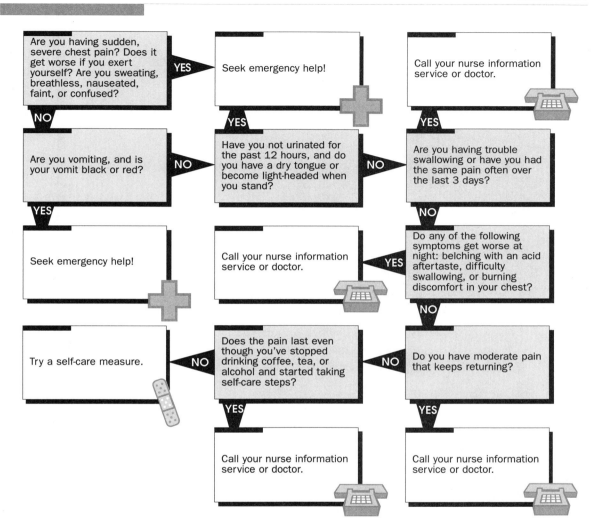

Are you having sudden, severe chest pain? Does it get worse if you exert yourself? Are you sweating, breathless, nauseated, faint, or confused?

YES → Seek emergency help!

NO ↓

Are you vomiting, and is your vomit black or red?

NO → Have you not urinated for the past 12 hours, and do you have a dry tongue or become light-headed when you stand?

YES ↓

YES → Call your nurse information service or doctor.

NO → Are you having trouble swallowing or have you had the same pain often over the last 3 days?

YES → Seek emergency help!

Call your nurse information service or doctor.

YES ← Do any of the following symptoms get worse at night: belching with an acid aftertaste, difficulty swallowing, or burning discomfort in your chest?

NO ↓

Try a self-care measure.

NO ← Does the pain last even though you've stopped drinking coffee, tea, or alcohol and started taking self-care steps?

NO ← Do you have moderate pain that keeps returning?

YES ↓

Call your nurse information service or doctor.

YES ↓

Call your nurse information service or doctor.

---

specific irritants or foods that are worst for you. The following general rules apply to everybody:

- Avoid problem foods.
- Straighten up your posture, both sitting and standing. Move around; walk. After eating, don't lie down or bend over. Prop up the head of your bed so gravity helps keep the stomach acid down, where it belongs.
- Lose weight if you are more than 20% over your ideal weight.

- Eat small meals and nothing for 2 to 3 hours before bedtime.
- Avoid foods that contain a lot of air (e.g., whipped cream) or carbonated drinks, and don't drink through a straw or from a narrow-necked bottle.
- Avoid tight clothing, especially around the waist.

HEEL PAIN

The Problem
Your heel hurts.

Causes of Heel Pain

Other Causes

Injury
Plantar fascitis
Calcaneal (heel bone) spur
(*see* page 98)
Rheumatoid arthritis
(*see* page 224)
Gout (*see* page 108)

Inflamed tendon. The soles of your feet hurt from the front of your heel up through the balls of your feet. The tendons in your feet, the tough, inelastic cords that connect muscle to bone, are prone to inflammation from overuse, sudden twists and turns, and repetitive stress from poorly fitting or unsupportive shoes that encourage poor foot positioning.

Bursitis. The fluid-filled sacs called bursae reduce the friction between tendon and bone. They can become inflamed from poor-fitting shoes that squeeze the bursae or from the pressure of landing hard on your heels, as after a high jump or unexpected backward fall. Self-care measures should help, although you may need a shoe insert to correct improper walking.

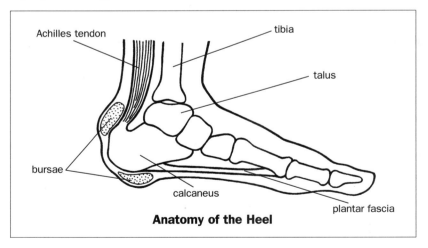

Anatomy of the Heel

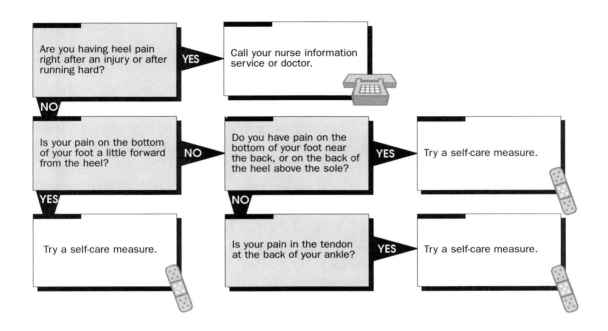

Are you having heel pain right after an injury or after running hard? **YES** → Call your nurse information service or doctor.

NO ↓

Is your pain on the bottom of your foot a little forward from the heel? **NO** → Do you have pain on the bottom of your foot near the back, or on the back of the heel above the sole? **YES** → Try a self-care measure.

YES ↓

Try a self-care measure.

NO ↓

Is your pain in the tendon at the back of your ankle? **YES** → Try a self-care measure.

Achilles tendinitis. The Achilles tendon, one of the strongest tendons in the body, connects the back of the heel to the muscles of the calf. When it becomes inflamed, perhaps with swelling and tenderness, it is often the result of strain on calf muscles that have become too tight through lack of stretching. Runners who jog on hard surfaces and athletes who wear unsupportive footwear are prone to Achilles tendinitis. Try a self-care measure.

Self-Care Measures

- All heel problems require a long time to correct. For an inflamed tendon, bursitis, fasciitis, or Achilles tendinitis, try the following:

– Rest your feet as much as possible for a week.
– Use aspirin or ibuprofen (*see* page 27) to relieve the pain.
– Wear proper shoes, heel pads, and arch supports.
– Ice massage for 5 minutes after walking.

Prevention

- Wear comfortable shoes every day. When exercising or working out, use proper footwear.
- Learn appropriate stretching and strengthening exercises for your feet and ankles.

HIP PAIN

The Problem

You have pain in the area of your upper thigh and lower buttock or in your groin area.

Other Causes

Osteoarthritis (*see* page 224)

Referred pain, especially from the back

Aseptic necrosis

Tendinitis (*see* page 174)

Rheumatoid arthritis (*see* page 224)

Structural defect

Ankylosing spondylitis

Polymyalgia rheumatica

Circulatory problem

Causes of Hip Pain

Hip fracture. You fell recently, and now you are experiencing a great deal of hip pain; when you lie down, you can't straighten your leg and raise it. The hipbone—actually the top of the leg bone—can break easily, even after only a slight fall. Most at risk are elderly people and those with osteoporosis (*see* page 250).

Excess body weight. You have chronic pain in your hip that worsens after you've been walking or standing for a prolonged period. The hip is a major weight-bearing joint, and the more weight it has to bear, the more painful it can become.

Bursitis. You have pain and tenderness in the area of your hip joint; it may spread down the leg to the knee or worsen at night when you lie on it. Bursitis is an inflammation of the bursae, the fluid-filled sacs that cushion the bony part of the hip and reduce the friction caused by movement.

Self-Care Measures

- Avoid activities that aggravate your hip pain. Pain is your body's way of telling you to slow down; don't ignore the message. You don't have to stop exercising entirely, but perform only stretching and non-weight-bearing exercises.

- Apply moist heat to your hip area for 20 minutes, 3 or 4 times a day. Use a towel soaked in hot water and wrung out (place a dry towel over the wet one to hold in the heat) or a moist heating pad.

Treating Your Child

- Don't give aspirin to anyone under 19 years of age! It may cause a rare but serious problem called Reye's syndrome. Instead, use ibuprofen or acetaminophen (*see* page 27) for fever or pain.

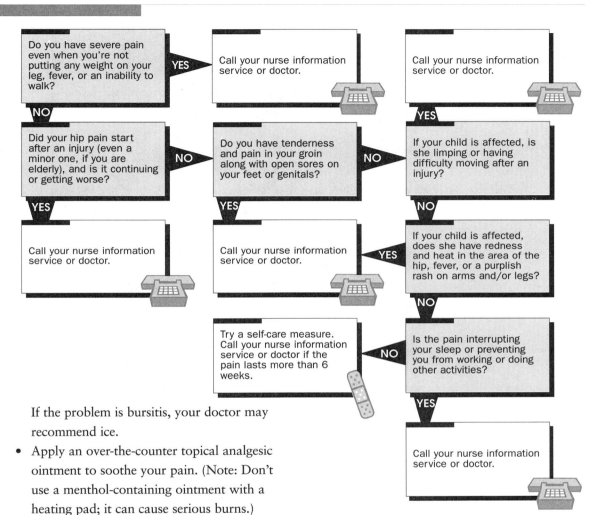

If the problem is bursitis, your doctor may recommend ice.

- Apply an over-the-counter topical analgesic ointment to soothe your pain. (Note: Don't use a menthol-containing ointment with a heating pad; it can cause serious burns.)
- Massage the area around your hip joint.
- Sleep on a firm mattress, preferably on your back. Avoid lying on the painful hip. Do not put pillows under your knees or lower back.
- Try an over-the-counter pain reliever such as aspirin, acetaminophen, or ibuprofen (*see* page 27).

Prevention

- Exercise is good, but too much can cause hip discomfort. If you have the beginnings of hip pain, try low-impact exercise, like swimming, bicycling, or walking. Buy running shoes—not walking, aerobic, or cross-training shoes—for walking; they are extra light and designed to increase the stability of the foot.
- Lose weight (*see* page 25). Even if your hip pain is not a direct result of being overweight, if you're carrying too many pounds, losing weight can take pressure off your hip and greatly decrease your pain.

HIVES

The Problem

You have raised, red, and probably itchy welts (i.e., ridges or bumps) on your skin. Hives usually appear on the face, arms, legs, or trunk of the body; less often, they occur on the scalp, hands, or feet.

Important Information About Hives

In the great majority of cases, hives are an *allergic* response to something you touched, inhaled, or swallowed. They form because histamine, a chemical that the body produces as part of the allergic response, causes fluid to leak out of the blood vessels and collect under the skin. Hives are more common in allergy-prone people who have hay fever, dust allergies, and eczema. It is difficult to determine the exact cause of most hive-producing allergies. However, the following are frequent offenders:

- Animal dander
- Berries
- Bug bites or stings
- Chocolate
- Dairy products
- Eggs
- Freshwater fish
- Medications
- Nuts
- Pollen
- Pork
- Shellfish
- Wheat products

In addition to allergies, hives can be caused by exposure to cold or heat, emotional or physical stress (including exercise), and, very rarely, *cancer* or connective tissue disease. Hives are usually harmless. They go away on their own, leaving no scars, and cause no lasting problems. In very rare cases, however, hives can be the first sign of a life-threatening allergic reaction called *anaphylaxis*. Without prompt treatment, airway obstruction, shock, coma, heart attack, and even death can occur.

Treating Your Child

- See *Self-Care Measures* and *Prevention* listed here.

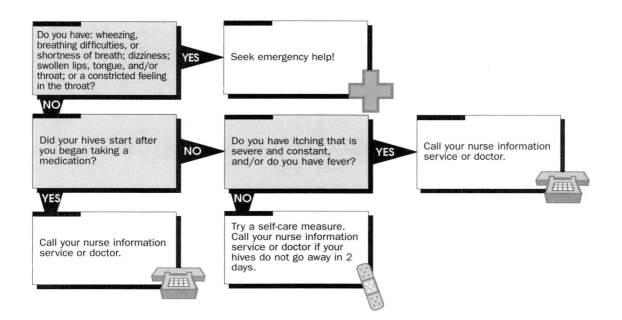

Do you have: wheezing, breathing difficulties, or shortness of breath; dizziness; swollen lips, tongue, and/or throat; or a constricted feeling in the throat?

YES → Seek emergency help!

NO ↓

Did your hives start after you began taking a medication?

NO → Do you have itching that is severe and constant, and/or do you have fever?

YES → Call your nurse information service or doctor.

YES ↓

Call your nurse information service or doctor.

NO ↓

Try a self-care measure. Call your nurse information service or doctor if your hives do not go away in 2 days.

Self-Care Measures

- Take cool (not even warm) showers. Cool water will ease the histamine reaction (hot water will stimulate histamine release and worsen your hives).
- Wear loose-fitting, lightweight clothing, especially if your hives are very itchy.
- Try an over-the-counter antihistamine. Keep in mind that these antihistamines can cause drowsiness and make it dangerous for you to drive or perform other activities requiring alertness. If that poses a problem, ask your nurse information service or doctor about possible prescription antihistamines that don't cause drowsiness. Do not drink alcoholic beverages while taking these drugs. If you are pregnant or a breast-feeding mother, do not take antihistamines unless your doctor recommends it.

- Avoid taking aspirin, ibuprofen, naproxen sodium (*see* page 27), or narcotics; these medications may aggravate hives.

Prevention

- If you've experienced an outbreak of hives more than once, try to identify the cause of the reaction. The substances listed above in "Important Information About Hives" are the most common culprits.
- Avoid diet drinks and foods with many additives, dusty places, and chemicals that come in contact with your skin (e.g., makeup, cologne, shampoo, and/or soap).
- Eliminate all possible allergen sources at once, and then reintroduce them one at a time in order to identify what's causing your hives.

125

HOARSENESS/LOSS OF VOICE

The Problem

Your voice is husky and raspy, and the problem may be so severe that you can barely make any sound at all.

Causes of Hoarseness and Loss of Voice

Other Causes

Heartburn (*see* page 118)
Dry air
Allergic rhinitis (*see* page 256)
Nodule
Cyst
Polyp
Anxiety or stress
Stroke (*see* page 258)
Throat *cancer*
Lung *cancer*
Multiple sclerosis
Amyotrophic lateral sclerosis
Parkinson's disease

Infection. You've become hoarse gradually over the past few days, and you also have, or recently had, a cold, a sore throat, a cough, and/or a fever. An upper respiratory tract infection leading to laryngitis (*see* page 196) is one of the most common causes of hoarseness. You can treat the infection and resulting loss of voice with self-care measures if the problem is caused by a virus. If you have a bacterial infection, however, you'll need antibiotics.

Overuse. You spent the afternoon cheering your favorite ball team to victory, and now your voice is hoarse and raspy. Using your vocal cords excessively, whether occasionally (e.g., yelling at the kids) or chronically (e.g., if you are a teacher or a singer), can cause laryngitis. Self-care measures, most importantly resting your vocal cords, should return your voice to normal within a week.

Irritant. You've spent an evening drinking and chatting with friends in a noisy, smoky bar, and now you can hardly talk, but you have no other symptoms. Alcohol in large amounts can irritate the vocal cords, and although there are other respiratory irritants, cigarette smoke is one of the worst. Cigarette smoke can also cause hoarseness by producing tumors on the vocal cords, a problem that affects smokers more than anyone else. If you smoke, quit (*see* page 24), and avoid exposure to secondhand smoke.

Treating Your Child

- A hoarse cry or inability to make any sound may indicate a serious problem in a child under 3 months of age, so call your nurse information service or doctor.
- If your child is under the age of 4 and has, in addition to hoarseness, a cough that sounds like a barking seal, the likely cause is croup, a common disease. Turn the shower on hot and full blast; then sit with your child outside the shower and let him inhale the steam. Or take a walk outside in the cold night air. A cool vaporizer close to the bed may also help. Typically, your child should feel better in the morning.

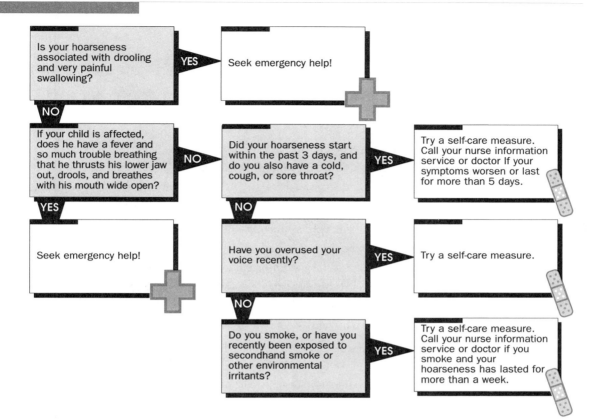

Is your hoarseness associated with drooling and very painful swallowing? — **YES** → Seek emergency help!

NO ↓

If your child is affected, does he have a fever and so much trouble breathing that he thrusts his lower jaw out, drools, and breathes with his mouth wide open? — **NO** → **Did your hoarseness start within the past 3 days, and do you also have a cold, cough, or sore throat?** — **YES** → Try a self-care measure. Call your nurse information service or doctor If your symptoms worsen or last for more than 5 days.

YES ↓

Seek emergency help!

NO ↓ (from "Did your hoarseness start within the past 3 days...")

Have you overused your voice recently? — **YES** → Try a self-care measure.

NO ↓

Do you smoke, or have you recently been exposed to secondhand smoke or other environmental irritants? — **YES** → Try a self-care measure. Call your nurse information service or doctor if you smoke and your hoarseness has lasted for more than a week.

Hypothyroidism. Your voice is hoarse, and you also notice that you're more sensitive to cold than you usually are, that your skin and hair are very dry, that you've gained weight without increasing your food intake, and that you're tired all the time. Hypothyroidism, or an underactive thyroid gland, is most likely to occur in middle-aged women. A blood test is needed to diagnose this condition, and you'll need to take synthetic thyroid hormone tablets to correct it.

Self-Care Measures

- Try not to use your voice. Speak as little as possible, and most importantly, avoid talking too loudly or softly. Whispering puts nearly as much stress on your vocal cords as shouting does.

- Inhale steam from a hot shower or from a vaporizer, and drink plenty of water (i.e., at least 6–8 glasses a day).

- Avoid aspirin; it can further irritate your vocal cords. If you have a sore throat along with your hoarseness and you're looking for pain relief, take acetaminophen (*see* page 27) instead.

- Avoid gargling. Most mouthwashes contain alcohol, which can irritate and dehydrate the mucous membranes. Moreover, the gargled liquid doesn't get anywhere near the vocal cords.

Prevention

- Avoiding irritants is the key to preventing hoarseness, so avoid cigarette smoke, as well as chemical fumes and wood dust.

- Try not to overuse your voice.

INCONTINENCE

The Problem

You often feel an urgent need to urinate, or you are unable to hold back urine, resulting in dribbling or leaking.

Other Causes

Chronic cystitis
Aging or senility
Diabetes (*see* page 240)
Nutritional deficiency
Medication side effect
Stroke (*see* page 258)
Spinal cord injury

Causes of Urinary Incontinence

Bladder infection. You have urgent, painful, frequent, not very productive urination with blood in the urine, a fever, and lower back and pelvic pain. Bladder infections, or cystitis, are among the most common causes of incontinence and are treated with antibiotics.

Prostate problem. You are having difficulty urinating, get up at night to urinate, and you urinate often but with less volume. This may be a minor prostate inflammation or enlargement that you should discuss with your doctor during your next visit. If you also have pain in the lower back and pelvic area and painful ejaculation or bowel movements, this may be an indication of a more serious prostate problem.

Estrogen deficiency. You are approaching or undergoing menopause (*see* page 206) and are having embarrassing episodes of leakage. Incontinence has been linked to decline in estrogen production by the ovaries, which leads to thinning of the tissues lining the *urethra*. Many women find local estrogen cream effective against leakage. You may wish to discuss hormone replacement therapy with your doctor during your next visit.

Self-Care Measures

- Use adult diapers or pads only if recommended by your nurse information service or doctor. You may need other treatment.
- Try to regain some control over your bladder by going to the bathroom often and regularly.
- Women can learn Kegel exercises to strengthen the pelvic floor muscles. Practice stopping urination in midstream and then starting

Treating Your Child

- See *Self-Care Measures* and *Prevention* listed here.

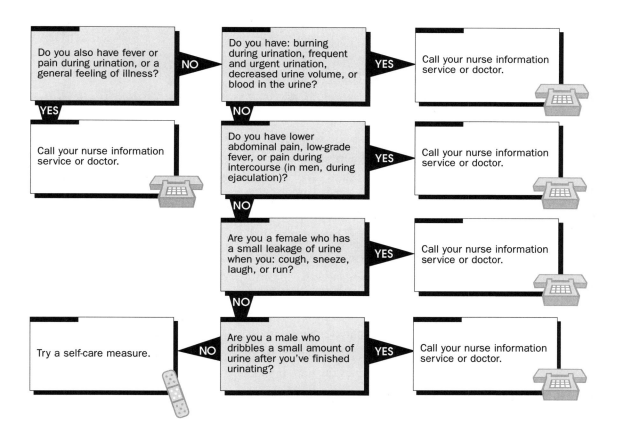

Do you also have fever or pain during urination, or a general feeling of illness?

NO → Do you have: burning during urination, frequent and urgent urination, decreased urine volume, or blood in the urine?

YES → Call your nurse information service or doctor.

YES ↓

Call your nurse information service or doctor.

NO ↓

Do you have lower abdominal pain, low-grade fever, or pain during intercourse (in men, during ejaculation)?

YES → Call your nurse information service or doctor.

NO ↓

Are you a female who has a small leakage of urine when you: cough, sneeze, laugh, or run?

YES → Call your nurse information service or doctor.

NO ↓

Try a self-care measure.

NO ← Are you a male who dribbles a small amount of urine after you've finished urinating?

YES → Call your nurse information service or doctor.

again. Contract the muscles around your vagina and anus, hold for a couple of seconds, then relax. Repeat. Do this throughout the day.

- Try double voiding: Empty the bladder as completely as possible. Then, a couple of minutes later, try to empty it again.

Prevention

- Avoid drinking anything between your evening meal and bedtime, especially alcohol and caffeinated drinks.

- Determine if any of your usual medications could be contributing to incontinence, and discuss a possible change in your medication with your nurse information service or doctor.

INSOMNIA

The Problem

You can't fall asleep, or you wake in the night and can't get back to sleep. The problem can last for days or months.

Causes of Insomnia

Other Causes

Anxiety or stress
Depression (*see* page 238)
Psychiatric disorder
Late evening exercise
Lack of regular exercise
Noise
Menopausal *hot flash*
Daytime napping

Caffeine, alcohol, or drug use. You drink coffee, tea, or cola drinks, or eat chocolate—probably to excess, but if you're sensitive, even small amounts of caffeine make you wakeful. You may be a smoker, or you're using over-the-counter decongestants, cold remedies, diet pills, or a bronchodilator before bedtime. Both sleeping pills and alcohol often make you feel sleepy but can lead to "rebound" insomnia (in which your body becomes dependent on sleeping pills or alcohol in order to sleep). The sleep induced by pills or alcohol may also be shallow and not restful.

Medical problem. You have chronic pain, especially if you are elderly and have joint disease. You may have *angina* (chest pain) or breathing difficulties (*see* page 48) because of heart-lung disease. If you snore, sleep fitfully, and are sleepy during the day, you may have sleep apnea (*see* page 72). Prostate trouble (*see* page 254), diabetes (*see* page 240), or a urinary tract infection may be the cause if your sleep is disturbed by the need for frequent urination. If you have *allergies* or respiratory ailments such as chronic obstructive pulmonary disease (*see* page 232), you may have trouble breathing when lying down, which keeps you awake. If you have restless leg syndrome, the twitching in your legs may wake you.

Self-Care Measures

- Stop struggling to sleep. If you don't fall asleep in 20 minutes, get up and do something to relax: read a book or a magazine, use a relaxation technique, and/or listen to relaxation or mood-softening tapes.
- Don't use alcohol to help you sleep; try warm milk instead.
- If you are experiencing hot flashes or night sweats, try using a fan on a low setting while sleeping. However, if the hot flashes are due to

Treating Your Child

- See *Self-Care Measures* and *Prevention* listed here.

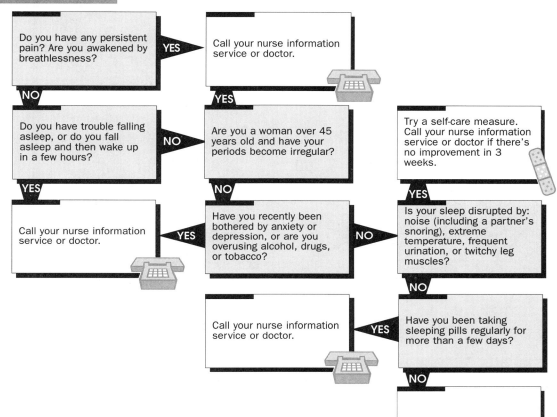

Do you have any persistent pain? Are you awakened by breathlessness? **YES** → Call your nurse information service or doctor.

NO ↓

Do you have trouble falling asleep, or do you fall asleep and then wake up in a few hours? **YES** ↓ **NO** → Are you a woman over 45 years old and have your periods become irregular? **YES** ↑ → Try a self-care measure. Call your nurse information service or doctor if there's no improvement in 3 weeks.

Call your nurse information service or doctor.

NO ↓

Have you recently been bothered by anxiety or depression, or are you overusing alcohol, drugs, or tobacco? **YES** ← **NO** → Is your sleep disrupted by: noise (including a partner's snoring), extreme temperature, frequent urination, or twitchy leg muscles? **YES** ↑

Call your nurse information service or doctor. ← **YES** Have you been taking sleeping pills regularly for more than a few days? **NO** ↑

NO ↓

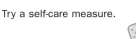

Try a self-care measure.

menopause (*see* page 206), call your nurse information service or doctor. You may need prescription medication.

Prevention

- Identify the cause; eliminate it or limit its effects.
- Don't use your bedroom for anything not associated with rest, sleep, or sex.
- Take a warm (not hot) bath or shower before bed.
- Don't eat for 3 hours before bed. At dinner, try cereal, bread, fruits, and foods rich in the sleep-inducing L-tryptophan (e.g., milk, turkey, and tuna fish).
- Don't smoke right before going to bed. Try to quit smoking (*see* page 24).
- Avoid caffeine during the day as well as at night. Remember that caffeine is found in diet aids and many cold/pain preparations as well as in coffee, tea, and chocolate.
- Don't go to bed if you're feeling wakeful and alert; but try getting up at about the same time every day, no matter what your bedtime was.
- Make your bedroom comfortable. Use clean sheets and pillowcases. Fresh air and darkness aid sleep. Avoid temperature extremes. Eliminate, reduce, or mask environmental noise.
- Don't exercise late in the evening.
- Avoid daytime napping.

JOCK ITCH

The Problem

You have itching, redness, and scaling in the groin area.

Causes of Jock Itch

Other Causes
Irritant

Fungal infection. Your groin itches after frequent visits to the gym or in other situations that may cause constant moisture in the groin area. You have an itchy, red, scaly rash on your groin. The fungus that has caused your jock itch thrives in warm, moist, dark places. Self-care and prevention are usually effective.

Pubic lice ("crabs"). These lice can be passed from one person to another by sexual contact or sometimes by contact with infested toilet seats, bed linens, or towels. Pubic lice look like little flakes of skin or dandruff.

Scabies. You have small, red blisters that itch severely. The itching may be worse at night or after a hot bath. Scabies is caused by tiny mites that burrow into your skin. Areas typically affected are wrists, armpits, elbows, ankles, soles of the feet, around the breasts and genitals, and on the buttocks. You may see tiny tracks that look like burrows. Blisters appear about 2 weeks after the mite has dug under your skin. Mites and eggs collected under your fingernails after scratching may be transmitted to other parts of your body. You can catch scabies from close physical contact with an infected person or from contaminated bedding or clothing. Over-the-counter and prescription treatments are available. Family members without symptoms should also be treated.

Medication side effect. You have recently started taking a new medication and you have itching in your groin area. Certain prescription and over-the-counter medications can cause itching as a

Treating Your Child

• See *Self-Care Measures* and *Prevention* listed here.

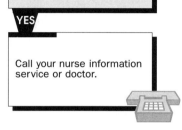

Is the itching severe and/or spreading from the groin to other parts of your body?

NO → Are your symptoms limited to the groin area?

YES → Try a self-care measure. Call your nurse information service or doctor if your symptoms last more than 2 weeks.

YES → Call your nurse information service or doctor.

side effect. Call your nurse information service or doctor and ask whether you need to switch medications.

Self-Care Measures

- Wash your groin gently, and blot dry with a towel (which should be laundered afterward), or use a hair dryer at its coolest setting.
- Try an over-the-counter antifungal remedy.
- Sleep naked or in loose fitting shorts.
- For scabies and pubic lice, use 5% permethrin cream, available over-the-counter. Follow the instructions on the packaging exactly. Before using the cream, take a bath or shower and scrub the affected area. Do not use on your

face. A second application may be necessary. Clothing and bedding should be washed in hot water. All members of your household should be treated, whether they have symptoms or not.

Prevention

- Keep your groin area clean and dry.
- Launder athletic supporters frequently.
- Don't leave damp underclothes in your locker or gym bag.
- Wear absorbent, loose, cotton underwear (including under your supporter during sports).
- Change clothes as soon as possible after sweating.

JOINT PAIN

The Problem

You have pain and/or stiffness in 1 or more of your joints (i.e., the soft tissue that joins bones and permits them to move).

Other Causes

Arthritis (*see* page 224)
Gout (*see* page 108)
Tendinitis (*see* page 174)
Bursitis
Infection
Lupus erythematosus
Hypothyroidism (*see* page 92)

Causes of Joint Pain

Injury. You have pain in 1 or more joints, and you've recently injured yourself in some way, perhaps in an automobile accident or by a sharp, sudden strain playing a sport. A common cause of injury is overuse (e.g., jogging or hiking), which may cause ankle (*see* page 32), knee (*see* page 136), or other lower-extremity pain. Self-help is useful for most joint injuries.

Self-Care Measures

- Apply ice to a fresh injury or to joint pain that has started recently. This will help keep the swelling down. The sooner you apply the ice, the better. You can use an ice pack, or you can make an ice wrap by using a 5-pound bag of frozen peas or corn. Apply the ice to your injury for 20 minutes; then leave it off for 20 minutes. Repeat this process at least 3 or 4 times a day for the first few days.
- Apply heat in the later stages of a joint injury or for pain you have had for some time. You can use a moist heating pad or hot water bottle, or you can make your own heating pad by putting a wet towel in the dryer and removing it while the towel is still damp and hot; place a dry towel over it to keep the heat in, and apply it to the injured area for 20 minutes; then leave it off for 20 minutes. Repeat this process 3 or 4 times a day.

Treating Your Child

- Don't give aspirin to anyone under 19 years of age! It may cause a rare but serious problem called Reye's syndrome. Instead, use ibuprofen or acetaminophen (*see* page 27) for fever or pain.
- If the joint pain did not follow an injury and your child has a fever and seems ill, call your nurse information service or doctor. Inflammation of the joint as a result of infection could be the cause of the pain, and your child may need antibiotics.

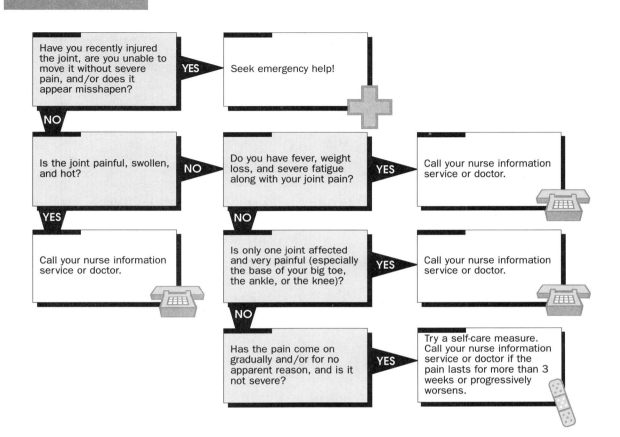

- Rest painful joints. If only 1 joint is painful, you can use a wraparound bandage or a brace to support and rest it. If several joints are involved, sit down, put your feet up, and rest for 15 minutes out of every hour.
- Try an over-the-counter pain reliever such as aspirin, ibuprofen, or naproxen with food (*see* page 27). They are particularly effective because of their anti-inflammatory properties, but alternating them with acetaminophen (*see* page 27) will be easier on your stomach.

Prevention

- Just as overuse can cause joint pain, underuse can cause it as well. Therefore, it's a good idea to get your whole body moving regularly, with a low-to-moderate-intensity exercise program. Swimming or walking in water (about chest-deep) is a particularly good activity when you have joint pain. This strengthens the muscles that cross the joints, making them more stable and less susceptible to further injury. The idea is to find a happy medium between rest and exercise.

KNEE PAIN

The Problem

You have pain and possibly stiffness and swelling in your knee. Since this large joint is designed to support the body's entire weight and is vital to your ability to move, significant disability can result from knee pain.

Other Causes

Sprain or strain (*see* page 182)
Arthritis (*see* page 224)
Tendinitis (*see* page 174)
Bursitis
Thrombophlebitis (*see* page 138)
Obesity (*see* page 248)
Infection
Foot problem
Tumor
Cyst

Causes of Knee Pain

Shin splints. You feel a gradual or sudden pain in the front and side of your lower leg during or after exercise. Shin splints result from repeated stress and pressure on the bones in the calf or the muscles or tendons surrounding it, and are common in anyone whose activity involves constant pounding of the feet on hard surfaces.

Post-traumatic effusion ("water on the knee"). Your knee aches and is very swollen. This condition results from an injury—a bang or a twist—that causes tissues in the knee to fill with blood and other fluids.

Dislocation. You've injured your knee within the last half hour and now have severe pain and swelling, and you have difficulty moving it. You may also be able to see that the knee is "out of joint."

Self-Care Measures

- If a sprain or strain is the cause, *see* page 182.

Treating Your Child

- Don't give aspirin to anyone under 19 years of age! It may cause a rare but serious problem called Reye's syndrome. Instead, use ibuprofen or acetaminophen (*see* page 27) for fever or pain.
- "Growing pains," which often center around the knee, are not unusual in children and adolescents. They result from plenty of physical activity, combined with the rapid muscle and bone growth that occurs during this period. Self-care measures can provide relief, but time is the best healer.
- Juvenile rheumatoid arthritis is a rare but possible cause of knee pain in children. In addition to joint pain, the symptoms include fever, rash, abdominal pain, weight loss, enlarged lymph glands, fatigue, and painful, red eyes. Call your nurse information service or doctor if you notice these symptoms in your child.

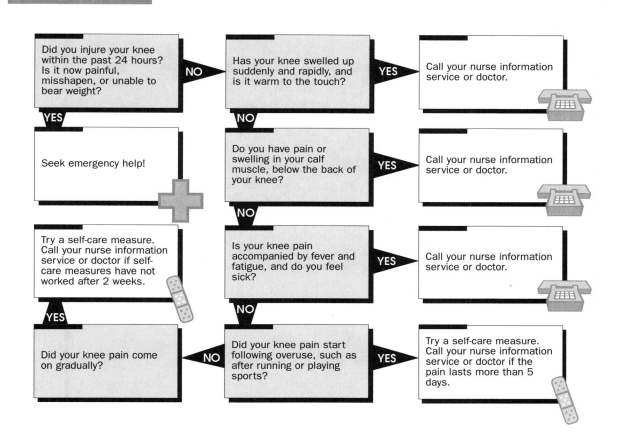

Did you injure your knee within the past 24 hours? Is it now painful, misshapen, or unable to bear weight?

NO → Has your knee swelled up suddenly and rapidly, and is it warm to the touch?

YES → Call your nurse information service or doctor.

YES → Seek emergency help!

NO → Do you have pain or swelling in your calf muscle, below the back of your knee?

YES → Call your nurse information service or doctor.

Try a self-care measure. Call your nurse information service or doctor if self-care measures have not worked after 2 weeks.

NO → Is your knee pain accompanied by fever and fatigue, and do you feel sick?

YES → Call your nurse information service or doctor.

YES → Did your knee pain come on gradually?

NO ← Did your knee pain start following overuse, such as after running or playing sports?

YES → Try a self-care measure. Call your nurse information service or doctor if the pain lasts more than 5 days.

- Try an over-the-counter pain reliever, such as aspirin, acetaminophen, or ibuprofen (*see* page 27). Aspirin and ibuprofen are best if your knee is also inflamed, but acetaminophen will be easier on your stomach if pain is your only symptom.
- Apply warmth—a hot water bottle; a moist heating pad; a warm, moist towel; or a warm bath—if your injury isn't recent or if you've had the pain for a few days.

Prevention

Anything that limits the amount of overuse and wear and tear that your knees get, especially the amount of weight they're forced to bear, can prevent knee problems.

- If you're overweight, try to lose a few pounds; even a small weight loss can make a big difference to the knees.
- If you spend long periods of time kneeling, cushion your kneecaps with protective knee pads or a cushion, and take frequent rest breaks so that the pressure isn't constant.
- Avoid squatting and find exercise alternatives to running; nonpounding activities, like swimming, walking, and biking, provide the same benefits but are much easier on the knees.

LEG PAIN/CRAMP

The Problem

You have pain in your thigh and/or calf. The pain may or may not last.

Causes of Leg Pain and Cramps

Cramp. You have sudden, severe pain in your calf or foot (especially at night and at rest), and you feel as though your muscle is in spasm; when you try to move the cramped muscle, it contracts violently, and the area feels hard and tense to the touch. As painful as they are, leg cramps are not serious. In almost all cases, there is no underlying cause—other than unaccustomed exercise or a prolonged period of sitting, lying, or standing in an awkward position—and no reason for concern.

Injury. Your leg pain came on suddenly, perhaps after a fall or after you hurt yourself while exercising. A severe injury, like a broken bone, can be distinguished from a less severe injury, like a muscle sprain or strain (*see* page 182), by determining whether you can bear weight on the leg: If you can't, the bone may be broken, and you'll need to seek emergency help. Muscle injuries, on the other hand, can be treated with self-care measures.

Superficial thrombophlebitis. You have a throbbing or burning pain in your calf, along with a feeling of heaviness; you may also notice that one of your veins is red and inflamed. Superficial thrombophlebitis—an inflammation of a vein located close to the skin's surface—is most likely to occur after a prolonged period of inactivity, such as extended bed rest or a long plane or car ride. Superficial thrombophlebitis is not a cause for concern, but it may be treated with anti-inflammatory drugs or blood thinners to prevent it from progressing into deep vein thrombosis (*see* page 32).

Other Causes

Sciatica
Arthritis (*see* page 224)
Varicose veins
Infection
Aneurysm

Treating Your Child

- Don't give aspirin to anyone under 19 years of age! It may cause a rare but serious problem called Reye's syndrome. Instead, use ibuprofen or acetaminophen (*see* page 27) for fever or pain.

- Toddlers can break their leg bones without sustaining an obvious, hard fall; an injury that simply twists the lower leg the wrong way can be enough to break the bone. Consider the possibility of a broken leg anytime your child is unable to bear weight on the limb following an injury.

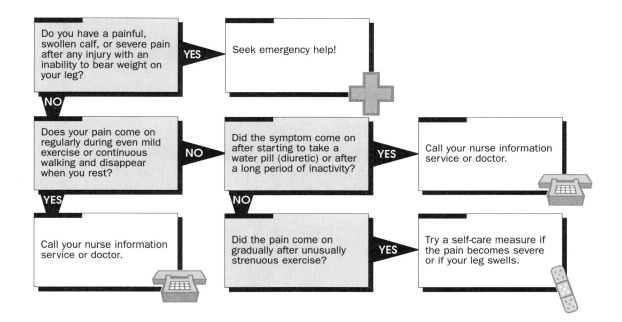

Intermittent claudication. You have a dull cramping feeling in your leg that comes on with exercise and goes away with rest. This problem is caused by a narrowing in the arteries of the leg, which prevents them from delivering enough blood to the muscles during even mild exercise. It is more common in older people and/or in heavy smokers. It is also often associated with the narrowing of arteries elsewhere in your body (especially the heart).

Self-Care Measures

- If a sprain or strain is the cause, *see* page 182.
- You can speed relief from sudden cramps by massaging and gradually stretching the cramped muscle.
- If your pain is due to superficial thrombophlebitis (your doctor must decide this), you can get some relief by lying down with your leg elevated and applying moist heat or a heating pad. Do not rub or massage the area.

Prevention

- Muscle cramps and spasms can often be prevented by warming up and stretching before exercising. In addition, make sure to drink plenty of water during exercise.
- Since intermittent claudication is caused by clogged blood vessels, the measures you need to take to prevent this pain will also help keep your heart healthy and prevent heart attacks: Stop smoking (*see* page 24), decrease your intake of high-fat foods (*see* page 17), and lose weight (*see* page 25).

LICE

The Problem

You are experiencing intense itching, and you notice some redness and flaking of your skin.

Important Information About Lice

Lice are tiny bugs, or parasites, that are about the size of sesame seeds. They pass easily from one person to another, and they survive by sucking human blood. They do not fly or jump, but they do crawl and can fall off their host. They die after 48 hours when detached from their host, and the eggs will not hatch if they fall off. Although annoying, they rarely pose a health risk.

Head lice. These are especially common in children, who pick them up at school, at day care centers, or at camp. They suck blood from the scalp, leaving red spots that may be extremely itchy. Because they are so small, it is difficult to see head lice; you're more likely to see the nits—small, pale eggs on the hair shafts, close to the scalp. They can pass from one person to another as long as they remain on the body and up to 24 hours after treatment.

Pubic lice ("crabs"). These lice can be passed from one person to another by sexual contact or sometimes by contact with infested toilet seats, bed linens, or towels. Pubic lice look like little flakes of skin or dandruff.

Body lice. These lice live in and lay their eggs on clothing and bedding, and only crawl onto the body when they need to feed. If you have body lice, you will notice itchy red spots no bigger than pinpoints. One to three itchy bumps clustered together may be caused by bedbugs, which are closely related to lice.

Treating Your Child

- Check your child for head lice at least once a week, especially during the peak season (i.e., August through November). Check more often if you notice frequent head-scratching.

- If your child has head lice, let close contacts know. Call friends' parents and the school or camp nurse. Treat your child with over-the-counter remedies, following the label instructions.

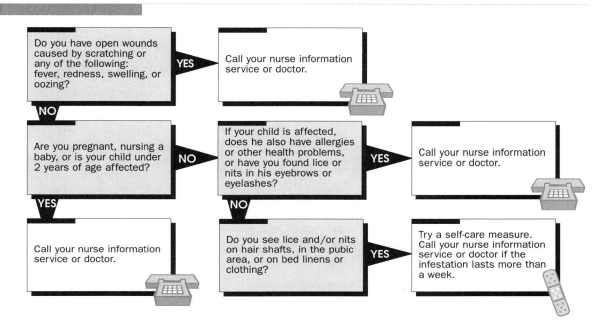

Do you have open wounds caused by scratching or any of the following: fever, redness, swelling, or oozing? — **YES** → Call your nurse information service or doctor.

NO ↓

Are you pregnant, nursing a baby, or is your child under 2 years of age affected? — **NO** → If your child is affected, does he also have allergies or other health problems, or have you found lice or nits in his eyebrows or eyelashes? — **YES** → Call your nurse information service or doctor.

YES ↓

Call your nurse information service or doctor.

NO ↓

Do you see lice and/or nits on hair shafts, in the pubic area, or on bed linens or clothing? — **YES** → Try a self-care measure. Call your nurse information service or doctor if the infestation lasts more than a week.

Self-Care Measures

There are many effective treatments available either by prescription or over the counter. Ask your nurse information service or doctor for a recommendation. Follow the package directions exactly; too much exposure to these products can be dangerous. Here are some other tips:

- It is essential to comb the hair repeatedly from the scalp outward using a fine-tooth comb dipped in hot vinegar until all lice and nits are removed.
- Soak all combs, brushes, and hair accessories for several hours in insecticidal shampoo or for 10 minutes in soap and hot water.
- Wash bedding and clothing in very hot water and dry on a high-heat cycle for at least 20 minutes. Heat kills the lice and destroys the nits.
- To kill lice in items that aren't washable, dry-clean them, or seal them in an airtight plastic bag. Don't open the bag for at least 2 weeks; then open it outdoors, and shake it vigorously.
- Thoroughly vacuum all mattresses, pillows, stuffed animals, rugs, and upholstered furniture. Dispose of the vacuum cleaner bag.
- If any family members have lice, all others must be treated (but call your nurse information service or doctor before treating anyone who is pregnant, nursing a baby, or under 2 years of age).
- If you have pubic lice, avoid sexual contact until you've completed treatment (*see* page 133). Any sexual partners in recent months should be informed.

Prevention

- Bathe and shampoo often.
- Avoid wearing the same clothing for more than 1 or 2 days.
- Change bed linens frequently.
- Do not share combs, brushes, hats, or headgear.

MOLE

The Problem

You have a small, roughly circular spot on your skin that is much darker than the skin surrounding it. It may be brown, black, or blue, and it may have coarse hair growing out of it.

Important Information About Moles

It is not known why people develop moles. They usually aren't present at birth, but develop as people get older. They often fade away on their own after many years. Most moles are completely harmless. Your risk of skin *cancer* is related to the amount of sun exposure you've had over your lifetime. Avoid excessive sun exposure whenever possible, and wear sunscreen when out in the sun. Moles have to be watched carefully, since *any* change in a mole could be a warning sign of melanoma (i.e., skin cancer). Use the **"ABCDE"** rule to determine if your mole is harmless or if it requires medical attention (*see* figure). Call your nurse information service or doctor if you notice any of the following:

Asymmetry. One half of your mole looks different than the other.

Border. The edges of your mole are ragged or irregular.

Color. Your mole has red, white, or blue patches, or a mixed brown or black color.

Diameter. Your mole is more than 1/4″ wide, or it has grown noticeably.

Elevation. Your mole has become raised.

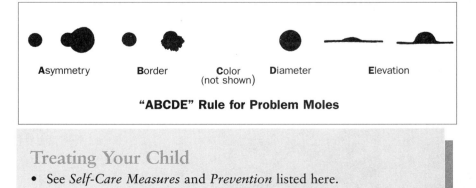

Asymmetry **Border** **Color** (not shown) **Diameter** **Elevation**

"ABCDE" Rule for Problem Moles

Treating Your Child

• See *Self-Care Measures* and *Prevention* listed here.

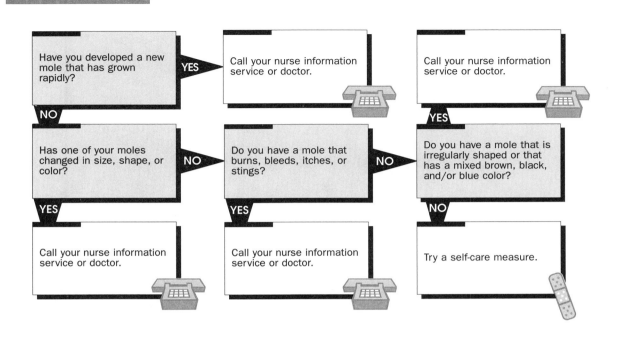

Have you developed a new mole that has grown rapidly? — **YES** → Call your nurse information service or doctor.

NO ↓

Has one of your moles changed in size, shape, or color? — **NO** → Do you have a mole that burns, bleeds, itches, or stings? — **NO** → Do you have a mole that is irregularly shaped or that has a mixed brown, black, and/or blue color? — **YES** → Call your nurse information service or doctor.

YES ↓

Call your nurse information service or doctor.

YES ↓

Call your nurse information service or doctor.

NO ↓

Try a self-care measure.

Self-Care Measures

- On a regular basis, examine your skin from head to toe. You're more likely to remember if you do it at a regular time (e.g., on the first day of each new season or month). Look for any changes in size, color, shape, or appearance of your moles. Use a hand mirror to check areas that you can't see easily.
- Be sure to have your skin examined by a health-care professional during physical examinations.
- Don't worry unnecessarily. If you do notice a change in a mole, it doesn't necessarily indicate skin cancer. If you're not sure, have the mole examined by a health-care professional just to be safe.

Prevention

- You can't prevent moles from forming. However, you should protect your skin by avoiding unnecessary exposure to the sun. Wear a hat with a wide brim and sunscreen with a sun protection factor (SPF) of at least 15 when outdoors.

MOUTH/TONGUE SORENESS

The Problem

You have a painful area (or areas) on your lips, on the insides of your cheeks, or on your tongue.

Causes of Mouth and Tongue Soreness

Other Causes

Vitamin B deficiency
Dry mouth (*see* page 46)
Gingivitis (*see* page 104)
Infection
Allergy
Salivary gland disorder
Leukoplakia
Oral lichen planus
Glossitis
Anemia (*see* page 90)
Neuralgia
Medication side effect
Oral *cancer*
Leukemia

Canker sore. You have a small, shallow, very painful sore on your lips, gums, inner cheeks, tongue, palate, or throat; it may be so painful that you find it hard to eat. You may have only 1 or as many as 10 to 15. Canker sores are extremely common, but it's not known what causes them. They are not dangerous, and they usually heal on their own within a few days to 2 weeks.

Cold sore. You have a painful sore on your lip (or perhaps inside your mouth) that started as a blister and has now ruptured. Cold sores, also called "fever blisters," are caused by the herpes simplex virus, and they are very common. They are uncomfortable and can be unsightly, but they are not dangerous, provided you don't touch the sores and then touch your eyes; doing so could cause a herpetic corneal ulcer. Cold sores are contagious, so avoid intimate contact. No treatment is required; they will go away on their own but usually recur.

Traumatic ulcer. You have a sore area inside your cheek or on your tongue, and you also have poorly fitting dentures or a broken, jagged tooth. Mouth sores can occur as a result of constant irritation and rubbing. You will need to correct the source of the problem in order to eliminate the sore.

Oral thrush. You have creamy yellow, slightly raised patches on the insides of your cheeks; if you rub them off when brushing your teeth or

Treating Your Child

- Infection with the Coxsackie virus, a very common and contagious virus in children, can cause mouth sores that are often accompanied by spots on the hands and feet (i.e., hand-foot-mouth syndrome). The child is likely to feel perfectly well and may or may not have a fever. The infection will clear up on its own within a few days to a week.
- Oral thrush (see above) occurs frequently in young children. It may clear up by itself, but it may require prescription treatment.

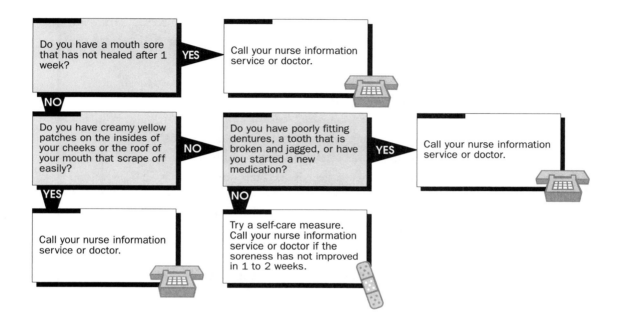

Do you have a mouth sore that has not healed after 1 week?

YES → Call your nurse information service or doctor.

NO

Do you have creamy yellow patches on the insides of your cheeks or the roof of your mouth that scrape off easily?

NO → Do you have poorly fitting dentures, a tooth that is broken and jagged, or have you started a new medication?

YES → Call your nurse information service or doctor.

YES

Call your nurse information service or doctor.

NO

Try a self-care measure. Call your nurse information service or doctor if the soreness has not improved in 1 to 2 weeks.

eating, they leave a painful, raw area. Oral thrush is caused by the fungus *Candida albicans*, one of the many microscopic organisms normally present in your mouth in small numbers. The bacteria in your mouth usually prevent this fungus from multiplying, but if your natural bacterial count drops (e.g., when you take antibiotics) or if your natural resistance to infection is low (as is seen with AIDS [*see* page 242]), this fungus may multiply out of control. You will require prescription treatment.

Self-Care Measures
- Drink plenty of water, and keep your mouth moist. Dry mouth itself can be a cause of mouth and tongue soreness, but it can also aggravate soreness caused by other factors.

- Do not smoke or chew tobacco. Smoking irritates the lining of your mouth, and chewing tobacco is even worse.
- Take a multivitamin supplement that contains vitamin C and the B vitamins.
- If it's painful to eat, cold liquids and ice pops can be soothing.

Prevention
- Keeping your teeth and gums in good condition with careful oral hygiene and regular dental visits can help prevent mouth sores.
- If you wear dentures, make sure that they fit, and get broken or cracked teeth fixed right away.

NAIL PROBLEM

The Problem

Your fingernail or toenail is discolored, split, thickened, crumbling at the edges, or pitted. You may have pain, swelling, and redness around a toenail.

Other Causes

Ingrown toenail (*see* page 198)
Paronychia (*see* page 96)
Finger or toe injury
Psoriasis (*see* page 66)
Illness

Causes of Nail Problems

Onychomycosis (fungal infection). Your nail is thick and yellow, with material building up under a slight separation at the end of your nail. If untreated, your entire nail may become separated, misshapen, or destroyed. Fungus affects fingernails only if they have been injured or if you have another skin disease; toenails can be infected without injury. You will require self-care and possibly prescription medication. It can take 6 months for fingernails to clear up and as long as 1 to 2 years for toenails.

Nail splitting. You have cracks along the nails or flaking at the ends. This is painless and may improve, but it may never disappear. Nail splitting tends to run in families, and it is sometimes caused by injury. Self-care is usually adequate.

Self-Care Measures

- If an ingrown toenail is the cause, *see* page 199.
- For an ingrown fingernail: Cut your nail straight across, not curving in at the corner. Push your skin back from the corner gently with a cotton swab twice a day. Keep the area clean.
- For blood under the nail: Bend open the end of a paper clip and heat the end over a lighter or gas stove. Be careful to hold the other end of the paper clip with an oven mitt or pliers so as not to burn yourself. Gently touch the hot tip to your nail, without pressing, and a painless hole will appear through which the blood can drain. This can be repeated, if needed, to relieve pressure.

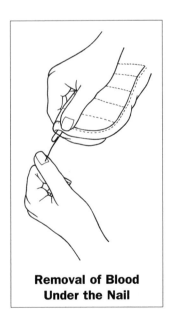

Removal of Blood Under the Nail

Treating Your Child

See *Self-Care Measures* and *Prevention* listed here.

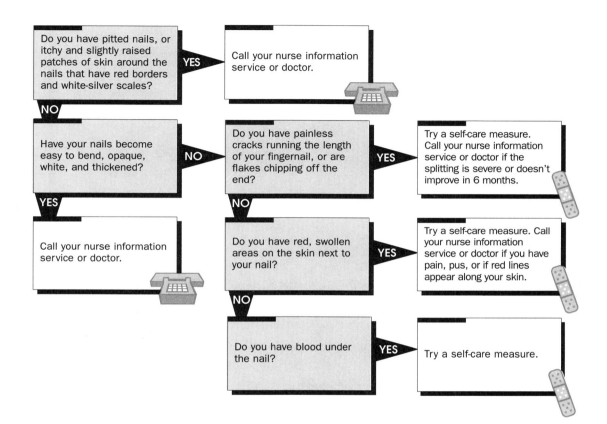

Do you have pitted nails, or itchy and slightly raised patches of skin around the nails that have red borders and white-silver scales?

YES → Call your nurse information service or doctor.

NO ↓

Have your nails become easy to bend, opaque, white, and thickened?

NO → Do you have painless cracks running the length of your fingernail, or are flakes chipping off the end?

YES → Try a self-care measure. Call your nurse information service or doctor if the splitting is severe or doesn't improve in 6 months.

YES ↓

Call your nurse information service or doctor.

NO ↓

Do you have red, swollen areas on the skin next to your nail?

YES → Try a self-care measure. Call your nurse information service or doctor if you have pain, pus, or if red lines appear along your skin.

NO ↓

Do you have blood under the nail?

YES → Try a self-care measure.

- For fungal infection: Dry your feet and hands thoroughly after bathing; use a hairdryer on its lowest setting to completely dry the nail. Go barefoot as much as possible, and avoid socks and shoes made of synthetics. Always wear cotton-lined latex or rubber gloves for dishwashing, cleaning, or any activity requiring your hands to be in water or chemicals. Avoid heat and excessive sweating. Over-the-counter remedies are usually ineffective.
- Nail splitting: Apply clear nail polish. Do not remove often. Wear cotton-lined latex or rubber gloves for cleaning. Rub hand cream on the skin around your nails.
- If paronychia is the cause, *see* page 96.

Prevention

- Keep your nails clean. Trim them weekly, clipping straight across; don't trim them too short (they should be at least roughly even with the tips of your fingers or toes). Avoid biting, picking, or tearing your nails or cuticles.
- Use nail polish remover sparingly; it dries your nails. Avoid nail strengtheners, artificial nails, and cuticle removers. They can discolor or break your nails, destroy the natural protection around them, and produce adverse reactions under your nails.

147

NAUSEA/VOMITING

The Problem

You feel queasy, as though you are about to throw up, and then you do. Vomiting is the actual expulsion of stomach contents due to sudden, forceful contractions of the muscles around the stomach; nausea is the sense that you are about to vomit.

Causes of Nausea and Vomiting

Other Causes

Medication side effect
Pregnancy
Gastritis
Motion sickness
Emotional upset
Migraine (*see* page 112)
Ulcer
Head injury (*see* page 110)
Meningitis (*see* page 150)
Appendicitis
Acute glaucoma (*see* page 230)
Hiatal hernia (*see* page 118)
Gallstones
Drug withdrawal
Bulimia

Gastroenteritis. You've had several bouts of nausea and vomiting, and you also have diarrhea, a headache, and a fever. Viral gastroenteritis, or viral infection, is the most common cause of nausea and vomiting in children and young adults. As miserable as it is, this condition usually passes on its own very quickly (often within 24 hours), although symptoms may last for as long as 5 days. Viral gastroenteritis can't be treated; it has to be allowed to run its course. But you can use self-care measures to help yourself feel better and to prevent *dehydration*, the most serious result of this condition.

Food poisoning. You are nauseated and vomiting, and you've recently eaten food that might have been spoiled (i.e., contaminated with bacteria). Many different kinds of bacteria can cause food poisoning. The nausea and vomiting usually start within 6 to 48 hours after eating the contaminated food, and these symptoms generally go away on their own within 1 to 2 days. Until then, self-care measures should be used to prevent dehydration.

Self-Care Measures

- The greatest danger with most vomiting is dehydration. If dehydration is a problem, *see* page 195.
- When you feel able to tolerate solids, start with bland, starchy

Treating Your Child

- Seek emergency help if you observe any of the following signs in a child who is vomiting: continuous abdominal pain for more than 3 hours, dry tongue, abnormal drowsiness, vomiting of greenish yellow matter.

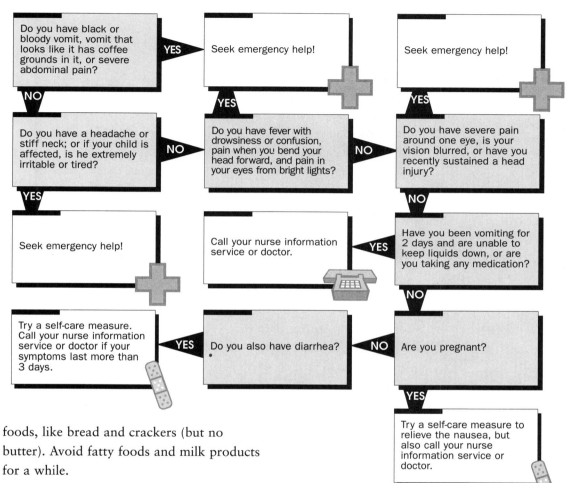

Do you have black or bloody vomit, vomit that looks like it has coffee grounds in it, or severe abdominal pain?

YES → Seek emergency help!

NO ↓

YES → Seek emergency help!

Do you have fever with drowsiness or confusion, pain when you bend your head forward, and pain in your eyes from bright lights?

Do you have a headache or stiff neck; or if your child is affected, is he extremely irritable or tired?

NO →

YES → Seek emergency help!

Do you have severe pain around one eye, is your vision blurred, or have you recently sustained a head injury?

NO ↓

YES ↓

Seek emergency help!

Call your nurse information service or doctor.

YES ← Have you been vomiting for 2 days and are unable to keep liquids down, or are you taking any medication?

NO →

NO ↓

Try a self-care measure. Call your nurse information service or doctor if your symptoms last more than 3 days.

YES ← Do you also have diarrhea?

NO → Are you pregnant?

YES ↓

Try a self-care measure to relieve the nausea, but also call your nurse information service or doctor.

foods, like bread and crackers (but no butter). Avoid fatty foods and milk products for a while.

- If pregnancy is the cause, try eating crackers or dry toast. Eat small, frequent meals throughout the day.

Prevention

- To prevent motion sickness, take an over-the-counter motion sickness medication at least an hour before you leave on your trip (but don't take these medications if you'll be driving; they can make you very drowsy). Ginger capsules (available in health food stores) also help without the side effects; take 3 or 4 capsules

(400-milligram) 15 minutes before you leave and every 4 hours thereafter.

- To prevent the nausea and vomiting associated with food poisoning, follow the rules of careful food preparation: keep hot foods hot and cold foods cold; wash your hands frequently while cooking; don't place any other food on a surface where raw meat has been; and cook all meats thoroughly (i.e., until the juices run clear).

NECK PAIN/STIFFNESS

The Problem

You have pain and/or stiffness in your neck.

Causes of Neck Pain and Stiffness

Other Causes

Arthritis (*see* page 224)
Prolapsed disk
Spinal cord damage
Heart attack (*see* page 54)
Cholecystitis
Peritonitis

Muscle strain and spasm. You have pain and stiffness in your neck, but you haven't sustained an injury recently, and you have no other symptoms. Muscle strain and spasm is the most frequent reason for neck pain. It can result from a wide variety of causes, including poor posture, emotional stress and tension (which can cause you to tighten your neck muscles for prolonged periods without even realizing it), or a recent or old neck injury. You can often find relief through self-care measures.

Pinched nerve. You have pain in your neck that extends down your arm and is limited to one side. You may also have numbness or tingling in your arm or hand. Arthritis (*see* page 224) or a neck injury can result in a pinched nerve in your spinal cord.

Meningitis. You have intense neck pain, accompanied by fever, severe headache, nausea/vomiting, drowsiness or confusion, and pain in your eyes when you look at bright lights. Your neck is so stiff that it is difficult to touch your chin to your chest. Meningitis is a rare but serious cause of neck pain.

Self-Care Measures

Since neck pain and stiffness are usually caused by muscle strain, there is much you can do to relieve them:

- Make sure the mattress you're sleeping on is firm. If you wake up with pain in the morning, sleep on a thin feather (not foam rubber) pillow, or try using none at all.

Treating Your Child

- Don't give aspirin to anyone under 19 years of age! It may cause a rare but serious problem called Reye's syndrome. Instead, use ibuprofen or acetaminophen (*see* page 27) for fever or pain.

- If your child has neck pain accompanied by fever, irritability, or lethargy, seek emergency help!

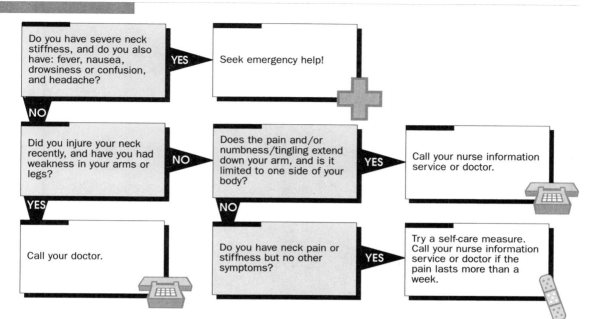

Do you have severe neck stiffness, and do you also have: fever, nausea, drowsiness or confusion, and headache?

YES → Seek emergency help!

NO ↓

Did you injure your neck recently, and have you had weakness in your arms or legs?

NO → Does the pain and/or numbness/tingling extend down your arm, and is it limited to one side of your body?

YES → Call your nurse information service or doctor.

YES ↓

Call your doctor.

NO ↓

Do you have neck pain or stiffness but no other symptoms?

YES → Try a self-care measure. Call your nurse information service or doctor if the pain lasts more than a week.

- For recurrent neck pain or pain that has continued for some time, try applying warmth (a moist heating pad or a warm, moist towel) to help loosen strained muscles. If your pain is from a recent injury, consult your nurse information service or doctor first.
- Try an over-the-counter pain reliever, such as aspirin, ibuprofen, or acetaminophen (*see* page 27) to relieve the pain. These remedies are generally as effective as prescription muscle relaxants for relieving neck pain and stiffness.

Prevention

- Improving your posture—not only when you sit and stand, but also when you move—can help to relieve neck pain and stiffness. Sit up straight and tall, raise your chest up, lower your chin slightly, and pull your head back so that your ears are directly over your shoulders.
- When you feel your muscles starting to tense up, take a break from what you are doing, massage your neck, rotate your head, and take deep breaths.

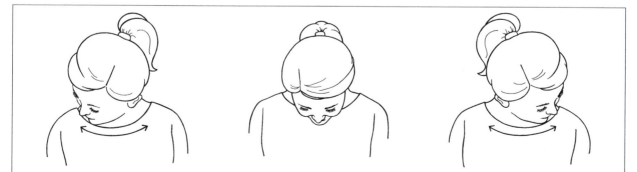

Loosen up your neck with exercise. Gently drop your head to your chest and then move it from one side to the other. Repeat several times.

NOSE, CONGESTED

The Problem

Your nose is stuffed up, you can't smell anything, and you may be able to breathe only through your mouth.

Other Causes

Allergic rhinitis (*see* page 256)
Common cold (*see* page 176)
Medication side effect
Decongestant spray use
Influenza
Sinusitis (*see* page 176)
Pregnancy
Polyp
Foreign body (*see* page 153)
Deviated septum

Causes of Nasal Congestion

Vasomotor rhinitis. You have a stuffy nose without itching and may have some nasal discharge; you are not sneezing. Nasal stuffiness can be relieved by avoiding humidity and changes in temperature. Overuse of nasal decongestants may make symptoms worse.

Self-Care Measures

- If sinus pain is the cause, *see* page 177. For an allergy, *see* page 257. If a common cold is the cause, *see* page 177.

Prevention

- If sinus pain is the cause, *see* page 177. For an allergy, *see* page 257.

Treating Your Child

- Don't give aspirin to anyone under 19 years of age! It may cause a rare but serious problem called Reye's syndrome. Instead, use ibuprofen or acetaminophen (*see* page 27) for fever or pain.
- If a foreign body is the cause, *see* page 153.

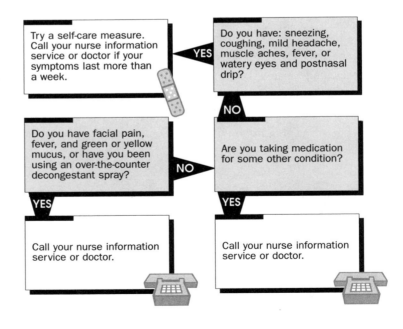

Try a self-care measure. Call your nurse information service or doctor if your symptoms last more than a week.

YES ← Do you have: sneezing, coughing, mild headache, muscle aches, fever, or watery eyes and postnasal drip?

NO ↓

Do you have facial pain, fever, and green or yellow mucus, or have you been using an over-the-counter decongestant spray? **NO** → Are you taking medication for some other condition?

YES ↓ Call your nurse information service or doctor.

YES ↓ Call your nurse information service or doctor.

NOSE, OBJECT IN

The Problem

You have a foreign object lodged in your nose.

Important Information About Objects in the Nose

Children tend to put or inhale things into their noses. Parents may not even be aware of a problem until the child complains of discomfort or sneezes a lot. If the object remains unnoticed for very long, the inner walls of the nose will become swollen, the nose will become stuffed up, and it may become infected with foul-smelling or bloody discharge.

Self-Care Measures

You must be extremely careful with self-care. Attempting to remove the object may cause it to be inhaled into the lungs.

- Do not try to move the object by poking at it with a swab or any other implement.
- Do not try to remove an object that has been in the nose more than several hours.
- Breathe through your mouth.
- Try to gently blow out through the affected nostril to dislodge the object, while holding the other nostril closed. Don't blow hard or more than a couple of times.
- If the object is visible and can be grasped with tweezers, try once to carefully remove it. If you are not successful, call your nurse information service or doctor.

Prevention

- Don't put small or sharp objects into your nose.

Treating Your Child

- Do not attempt to remove an object from a child's nose. Instead, call your nurse information service or doctor.

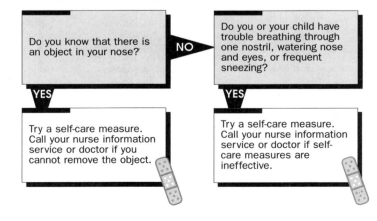

Do you know that there is an object in your nose?

NO → Do you or your child have trouble breathing through one nostril, watering nose and eyes, or frequent sneezing?

YES — Try a self-care measure. Call your nurse information service or doctor if you cannot remove the object.

YES — Try a self-care measure. Call your nurse information service or doctor if self-care measures are ineffective.

NOSE, RUNNY

Treating Your Child

- Don't give aspirin to anyone under 19 years of age! It may cause a rare but serious problem called Reye's syndrome. Instead, use ibuprofen or acetaminophen (*see* page 27) for fever or pain.

The Problem

Your nose is runny.

Causes of Runny Nose

Hay fever. You have a stuffy or runny nose, itchy eyes, and sneezing, but no other signs of illness. This is probably an *allergy*. Self-care measures can help.

Self-Care Measures

- If a cold is the cause, *see* page 177. For an allergy, *see* page 257. If sinusitis is the cause, *see* page 257.

Prevention

- Identify and eliminate allergens. Dress warmly in cool or cold weather. Wash your hands frequently. Drink at least 6 to 8 glasses of fluids every day.

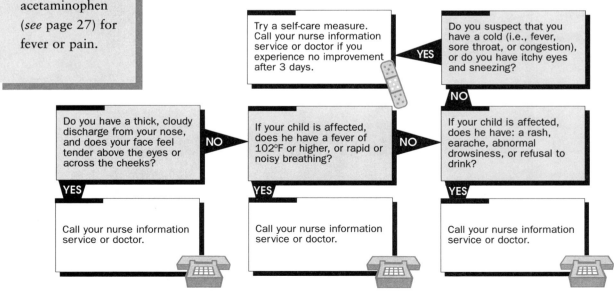

Do you suspect that you have a cold (i.e., fever, sore throat, or congestion), or do you have itchy eyes and sneezing? **YES** → Try a self-care measure. Call your nurse information service or doctor if you experience no improvement after 3 days.

NO ↓

If your child is affected, does he have: a rash, earache, abnormal drowsiness, or refusal to drink? **NO** ← If your child is affected, does he have a fever of 102°F or higher, or rapid or noisy breathing? **NO** ← Do you have a thick, cloudy discharge from your nose, and does your face feel tender above the eyes or across the cheeks?

YES ↓ Call your nurse information service or doctor.

YES ↓ Call your nurse information service or doctor.

YES ↓ Call your nurse information service or doctor.

NOSEBLEED

Other Causes

Hypertension (*see* page 244)
Hemophilia (*see* page 40)
Tumor
Blood vessel disease (*see* page 51)
Blood platelet disorder
  (*see* page 50)
Anticoagulant therapy
Dry air
Allergy
Aspirin use
Picking
Cocaine use
Blood clotting disorder
Leukemia

Treating Your Child

- See *Self-Care Measures* and *Prevention* listed here.

The Problem

Your nose is bleeding.

Causes of Nosebleeds

Injury. Your nose bled profusely for a while after you received a blow to the nose or head, but stopped after you applied self-care measures. Now your nose is oozing blood or clear fluid, is swollen, and may look crooked or misshapen.

Self-Care Measures

- Sit quietly with your head in a normal, upright position. Firmly pinch your nose shut by squeezing the septum (i.e., the inner divider just below the bone). Hold your nose shut constantly for 15 minutes. Breathe through your mouth.

Prevention

- If you are experiencing frequent nosebleeds, try using a humidifier to moisten the air and apply petroleum jelly to the inside lining of your nose once or twice a day; avoid aspirin, NSAIDs, and overuse of steroidal nose sprays.

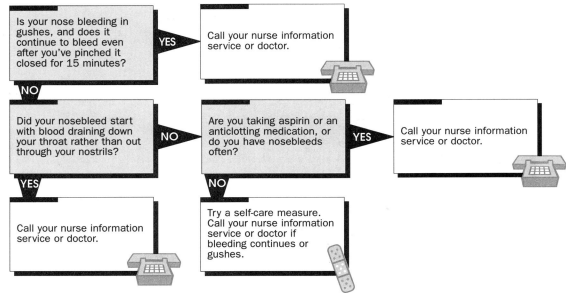

Is your nose bleeding in gushes, and does it continue to bleed even after you've pinched it closed for 15 minutes?
— YES → Call your nurse information service or doctor.
— NO

Did your nosebleed start with blood draining down your throat rather than out through your nostrils?
— NO → Are you taking aspirin or an anticlotting medication, or do you have nosebleeds often?
    — YES → Call your nurse information service or doctor.
    — NO → Try a self-care measure. Call your nurse information service or doctor if bleeding continues or gushes.
— YES → Call your nurse information service or doctor.

NUMBNESS/TINGLING

The Problem

You have no feeling in part of your body (it's "asleep"), or you have a pins and needles sensation.

Other Causes

Excessive cold
Circulatory problem
Rheumatoid arthritis
  (*see* page 224)
Diabetes (*see* page 240)

Causes of Numbness and Tingling

Nerve or blood vessel compression. You've been sitting in an awkward position or leaning or sleeping on one part of your body for too long. When you move, the numbness goes away, usually after some prickly tingling as the body part "wakes up." Leaning on your elbow may compress the ulnar nerve (i.e., your "funny bone"), causing tingling and numbness in your fourth and fifth fingers.

Carpal tunnel syndrome. The numbness and tingling in your hands (from thumb to ring finger) and wrists often get worse at night, and your fingers, thumb, and hand may be weak. You may be a constant user of certain power tools or computers or engage in other activities requiring repetitive motion. The condition may clear up by itself, or you may need anti-inflammatory drugs and a wrist splint.

Raynaud's disease. Your fingers and toes get numb and turn white, then blue, in cold weather and become red and painful when they warm up. You have a disorder of the small blood vessels.

Cervical osteoarthritis. You have numbness and tingling in part of your hands. You are probably over 50, and your neck is sometimes stiff and painful. You may have cervical osteoarthritis. If your neck pain spreads to your shoulders, the numbness and tingling move into your arms, and you walk unsteadily, you may have cervical *spondylosis*.

Herniated disk. You have lower back pain that worsens with movement, and you may feel pain, numbness, or tingling in your buttocks or legs. A herniated disk, or slipped disk, is a protrusion of the central part of one of the flat, circular pads found in the joints between the bones of the spine. Back injury, muscle weakness, or obesity (*see* page 248) is often the cause.

Treating Your Child

- See *Self-Care Measures* and *Prevention* listed here.

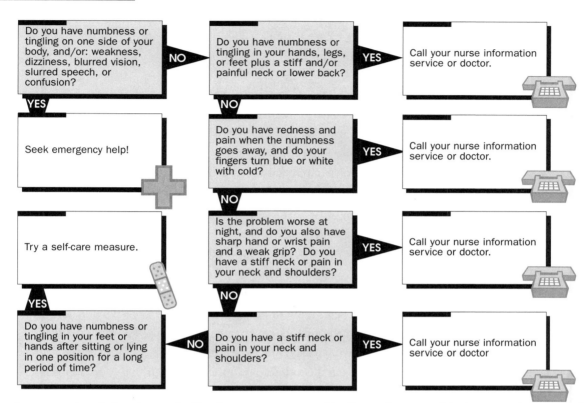

Do you have numbness or tingling on one side of your body, and/or: weakness, dizziness, blurred vision, slurred speech, or confusion? **NO** → Do you have numbness or tingling in your hands, legs, or feet plus a stiff and/or painful neck or lower back? **YES** → Call your nurse information service or doctor.

YES ↓

Seek emergency help!

NO ↓ Do you have redness and pain when the numbness goes away, and do your fingers turn blue or white with cold? **YES** → Call your nurse information service or doctor.

Try a self-care measure.

NO ↓ Is the problem worse at night, and do you also have sharp hand or wrist pain and a weak grip? Do you have a stiff neck or pain in your neck and shoulders? **YES** → Call your nurse information service or doctor.

YES ↓

Do you have numbness or tingling in your feet or hands after sitting or lying in one position for a long period of time? **NO** → Do you have a stiff neck or pain in your neck and shoulders? **YES** → Call your nurse information service or doctor

Stroke or transient ischemic attack. You have numbness and tingling on one side of your body with or without weakness in your arms or legs, slurred speech, blurred or double vision, confusion, and dizziness. These are warning signs of a transient ischemic attack or a stroke.

Self-Care Measures

- Massage the numb area to restore circulation.
- Move the limb or body part.
- Loosen your clothing.
- For Raynaud's disease, warm your hands and/or feet.
- If you have a slipped disk, lie on a firm surface with a small pillow under the knees or on your side with a pillow between your knees. Lie on a heating pad.

- Try ibuprofen or aspirin (*see* page 27) for neck or back stiffness.

Prevention

- Avoid sitting, leaning, or lying in one position for too long.
- Sit and stand correctly. Good posture will help to relieve pressure on your spine and neck. Sit up straight and tall, raise your chest up, lower your chin slightly, and pull your head back so that your ears are directly over your shoulders.
- Quit smoking. It impairs your circulation (*see* page 24).
- Break up repetitive tasks with rest or a change of task.
- Be sure your keyboard workstation allows optimal hand, wrist, and arm positioning.

PENIS PAIN/SWELLING

The Problem
Your penis is painful or sore.

Causes of Penis Pain and Swelling

Other Causes
Sexually transmitted disease
  (*see* page 202)
Allergy
Sports injury
Friction from clothing

Paraphimosis. Your uncircumcised foreskin has become retracted behind the head of your penis such that it cannot be brought forward. The swelling is severe. This condition may be treated by antibiotics or by a partial or complete circumcision (called a dorsal slit).

Balanitis. The tip of your penis is inflamed and irritated. This may be caused by a fungal or bacterial infection or an irritation from chemicals (such as dry-cleaning solvents in clothing). It occurs most frequently in men who are uncircumcised or have diabetes. You may need to take antibiotics, have your glans cleaned, and apply a soothing ointment.

Priapism. You have an erection that lasts for no apparent reason and is unrelated to sexual desire or activity. It is usually caused by a sudden, often unexplained obstruction that won't allow the blood that stiffens the penis to drain. Sometimes the cause is disease or injury of the spinal cord nerves, a gland condition, or a medication. If this condition is not treated promptly, erection could become permanently impossible.

Cancer. You had a small, painless, pimplelike growth (which you may not have noticed if you're uncircumcised) that is now a bleeding or oozing lump. Urinating may be painful, and you have lumps in your groin. Cancer of the penis is rare; it's often curable, but only with early diagnosis.

Self-Care Measures

- Most causes of penile pain should not be self-treated. For example, it is not advisable to try to force the foreskin to its normal place if it's painful or swollen, or to try to clean under it if it is irritated.
- If you have pain only during or after intercourse, it might be caused

Treating Your Child
- See *Self-Care Measures* and *Prevention* listed here.

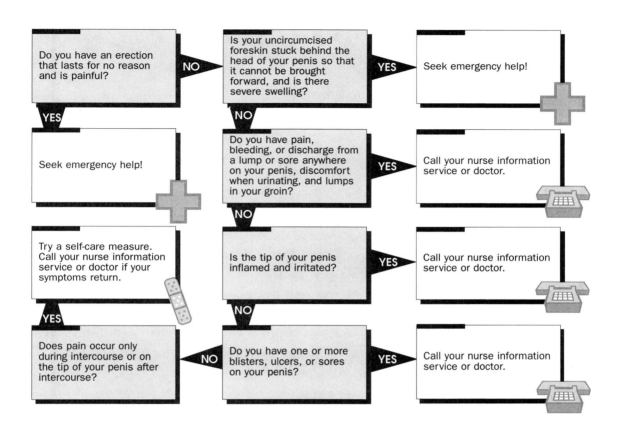

Do you have an erection that lasts for no reason and is painful?

NO → Is your uncircumcised foreskin stuck behind the head of your penis so that it cannot be brought forward, and is there severe swelling?

YES → Seek emergency help!

YES ↓

Seek emergency help!

NO ↓

Do you have pain, bleeding, or discharge from a lump or sore anywhere on your penis, discomfort when urinating, and lumps in your groin?

YES → Call your nurse information service or doctor.

Try a self-care measure. Call your nurse information service or doctor if your symptoms return.

NO ↓

Is the tip of your penis inflamed and irritated?

YES → Call your nurse information service or doctor.

YES ↓

Does pain occur only during intercourse or on the tip of your penis after intercourse?

NO ← Do you have one or more blisters, ulcers, or sores on your penis?

YES → Call your nurse information service or doctor.

by your partner's vaginal dryness. Lubricants and longer foreplay can help.

- If you have soreness in the tip of your penis after intercourse and are using latex condoms, try a nonlatex condom or another form of contraception. If the pain disappears, you're probably allergic to latex. Remember that nonlatex condoms do not protect against sexually transmitted diseases, including the HIV virus.

Prevention

- Minor irritations and inflammations can often be avoided by careful hygiene, especially after sexual activity and if you are uncircumcised. No special care, other than washing with soap and water, is needed.

159

RASH

The Problem

Your skin is red, spotty, blotchy, bumpy, scaly, rough, and/or blistered. It may itch or burn.

Other Causes

Diaper rash (*see* page 162)
Insect bite or sting (*see* page 184)
Hives (*see* page 124)
Fungal infection
Ringworm (*see* page 106)
Herpes (*see* page 42)
Shingles
Psoriasis (*see* page 66)
Lupus erythematosus
Meningitis (*see* page 150)
Kaposi's sarcoma (*see* page 243)

Causes of Rash

Allergy. You have raised red bumps with pale centers. Your skin may itch. Outbreaks can be caused by allergic reactions to food, or to something that comes in contact with the skin, including detergents, dry-cleaning solvents, fragrances, cosmetics, jewelry, plants (e.g., poison oak or ivy), wool, or latex gloves. Almost all drugs can cause allergic reactions.

Infection. You may have chicken pox, rubeola, rubella, fifth disease, or scarlet fever. Your rash can appear as a fine, sandpapery reddening or as red, black, or purplish spots that either fade to a flat, lacy pattern or become raised, like pimples. The rash starts on your face, abdomen, arms, or legs but usually spreads to the rest of your body. An infected child will have a fever, sore throat, and runny nose, and seem sick. Impetigo is a more localized infection that causes sores with a honey-colored crust.

Lyme disease. You've been bitten by a tick, and now you have a bull's-eye rash and one or more of the following: aching muscles, fever, fatigue, swelling of the knees or other joints, shortness of breath, temporary facial paralysis, heart irregularities, and/or memory and concentration problems.

Rocky Mountain spotted fever. You've been bitten by a tick, and now you have a severe headache, a fever of 103°F or higher, severe muscle aches and weakness, and a rash.

Treating Your Child

- Chicken pox: Give your child plenty of fluids. Use calamine lotion for itching. Bathe in cool water with baking soda or colloidal oatmeal (but no soap) every 3 or 4 hours for the first few days. Trim fingernails. Wash his hands 3 times a day with antibacterial soap. If there are sores in your child's mouth, eliminate salty or acidic foods. If diagnosed in the first 24 hours, a drug such as acyclovir can be helpful. There is now a chicken pox vaccine that is recommended for all children 12 months or older.
- Spray tick repellent on your child's clothes, but not on the skin.

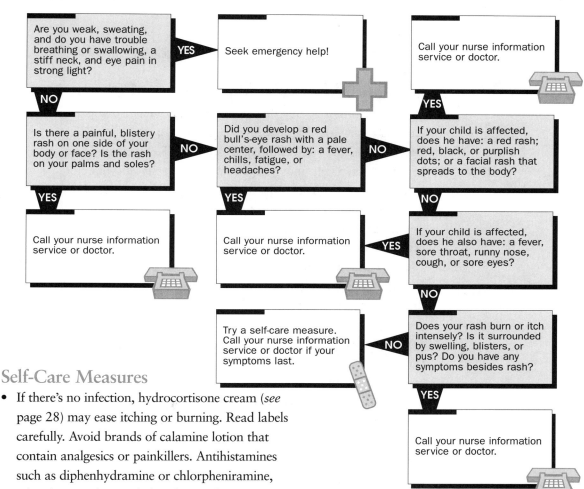

Are you weak, sweating, and do you have trouble breathing or swallowing, a stiff neck, and eye pain in strong light?

YES → Seek emergency help!

NO ↓

Is there a painful, blistery rash on one side of your body or face? Is the rash on your palms and soles?

NO → Did you develop a red bull's-eye rash with a pale center, followed by: a fever, chills, fatigue, or headaches?

YES ↓

Call your nurse information service or doctor.

Did you develop a red bull's-eye rash... **YES** ↓

Call your nurse information service or doctor.

NO → If your child is affected, does he have: a red rash; red, black, or purplish dots; or a facial rash that spreads to the body?

Call your nurse information service or doctor.

YES ↑

NO ↓

If your child is affected, does he also have: a fever, sore throat, runny nose, cough, or sore eyes?

YES → Call your nurse information service or doctor.

NO ↓

Does your rash burn or itch intensely? Is it surrounded by swelling, blisters, or pus? Do you have any symptoms besides rash?

NO → Try a self-care measure. Call your nurse information service or doctor if your symptoms last.

YES ↓

Call your nurse information service or doctor.

Self-Care Measures

- If there's no infection, hydrocortisone cream (*see* page 28) may ease itching or burning. Read labels carefully. Avoid brands of calamine lotion that contain analgesics or painkillers. Antihistamines such as diphenhydramine or chlorpheniramine, taken by mouth, may help relieve itching. Do not use antihistamines if you have glaucoma, heart, or prostate problems, or if you are pregnant or breast-feeding without first calling your nurse information service or doctor.
- For heat rash, take frequent cool baths without soap; air-dry. Use calamine lotion, but no oily ointments or creams.
- Wash poison ivy or oak rash quickly with soap and water (not hot) as soon as exposure occurs and for 2 or 3 days thereafter. Apply loose cold compresses. Soak often in cool water or bathe with lukewarm water and cornmeal.
- To remove ticks: With tweezers, grasp the tick as closely to your skin as you can; try to grasp the head as well. Pull slowly and evenly, straight up.

Prevention

- Check pets for fleas, and avoid areas where insects are found (*see* page 185). Try to identify and eliminate irritants or allergens. Avoid synthetic fabrics and cut down on laundry additives, such as softeners and bleaches; rinse twice.

RASH, DIAPER

The Problem
Your baby has red, spotty, moist, sore skin in the diaper area.

Important Information About Diaper Rash
Diaper rash is skin irritation that results from prolonged dampness and the contact of urine and feces with skin. Most babies will experience diaper rash at some point. Although infrequent diaper changes can make diaper rash more likely and more difficult to clear up, they are not necessarily the cause. Your baby may just have sensitive skin; often this rash goes away without treatment. Simple diaper rash can be complicated by infection with fungi or bacteria. When fungi are the culprit, the rash may have a tendency to recur. If the cysts are large and filled with liquid, the rash was caused by bacteria. Diaper rash can also occur in older children or in adults who wear diapers because of incontinence (*see* page 128).

Self-Care Measures
- If diaper rash is accompanied by a fungal infection (i.e., bright red rash, distinct border, and/or red patches outside the diaper area), use a topical over-the-counter antifungal cream.
- Keep the area as dry as possible. Change diapers frequently.
- Expose your baby's bottom to the air as much as you can. After a diaper change, try leaving the diaper off and placing your baby on a plastic sheet covered by soft towels. Do this frequently and for as long as possible, such as during a nap.
- Avoid using plastic pants. Use absorbent, disposable diapers until the rash clears.
- Do not use baby wipes; they may contain alcohol, which will further irritate the skin. Instead, use a clean, soft cloth moistened with clear, lukewarm water. Pat dry.

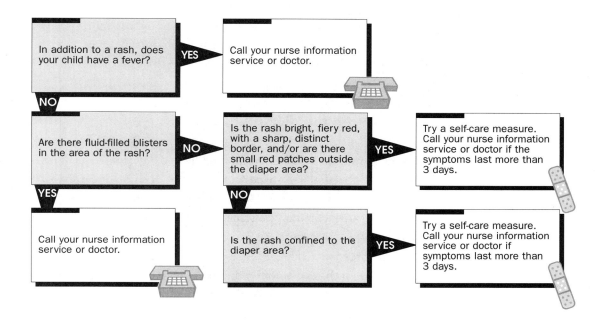

In addition to a rash, does your child have a fever?

YES → Call your nurse information service or doctor.

NO ↓

Are there fluid-filled blisters in the area of the rash?

NO → Is the rash bright, fiery red, with a sharp, distinct border, and/or are there small red patches outside the diaper area?

YES → Try a self-care measure. Call your nurse information service or doctor if the symptoms last more than 3 days.

YES ↓

Call your nurse information service or doctor.

NO ↓

Is the rash confined to the diaper area?

YES → Try a self-care measure. Call your nurse information service or doctor if symptoms last more than 3 days.

- Do not use cornstarch-based powder; it promotes the growth of fungal organisms.
- Bathe your baby each day in a tub with a gentle soap. Tub soaks after bowel movements, using mild soap and lukewarm water, can also help. Dry gently after washing.
- Squeezing the contents of vitamin E capsules over the affected area may help.
- If diaper rash occurs after several episodes of diarrhea, apply a thin layer of an over-the-counter petroleum- or zinc-based ointment or cream to protect the baby's skin.
- If you are using cloth diapers, when laundering, double rinse, and avoid using softeners.

Prevention

- Keep your baby as clean and dry as possible.
- Change your baby's diaper frequently.
- Expose his skin to the air whenever convenient.
- Do not use plastic pants. Use absorbent, disposable diapers.

RECTAL BLEEDING

The Problem

You notice blood in the toilet, on your toilet paper, or in your stool after you have a bowel movement. The blood may be bright red, or it may be burgundy-colored or black. (Be aware that bismuth-containing medications, like antidiarrheals, or iron supplements can cause black stools, and eating beets can cause red stools.)

Causes of Rectal Bleeding

Other Causes

Ulcerative colitis
Polyp
Anal warts (*see* page 212)
Crohn's disease
Proctitis
Diverticular disorder
Hemophilia (*see* page 40)

Hemorrhoids. You notice bright red blood on the toilet paper, in the toilet bowl, or on the stool itself after you have a bowel movement (as opposed to dark red blood mixed with the stool); you may also have pain during bowel movements. Hemorrhoids (sometimes called "piles") are by far the most common cause of rectal bleeding. They occur when the network of veins around the anus (i.e., the opening to the rectum) becomes engorged and enlarged. They are especially common during pregnancy and in those who often find themselves straining to have a bowel movement. Hemorrhoids can sometimes protrude through the anal opening, or they can be inside and invisible. The pain and inflammation usually disappear by themselves within a few days or weeks, but self-care measures can help in the meantime. If the pain and/or bleeding is severe and doesn't go away, call your nurse information service or doctor. Surgical treatment is an option but is rarely necessary.

Fissure. You notice bright red blood in your stool or on your toilet paper, and you have itching, along with pain, during and immediately after bowel movements. Anal fissures are crack-like sores that develop

Treating Your Child

- Small amounts of rectal bleeding and mild discomfort are common in babies or children with good appetites. The normal, frequent yellow stools of an infant can irritate the skin around and in the anus. In a young child, constipation is frequently the cause. Pinworms typically cause anal itching, and, very rarely, a little bleeding.

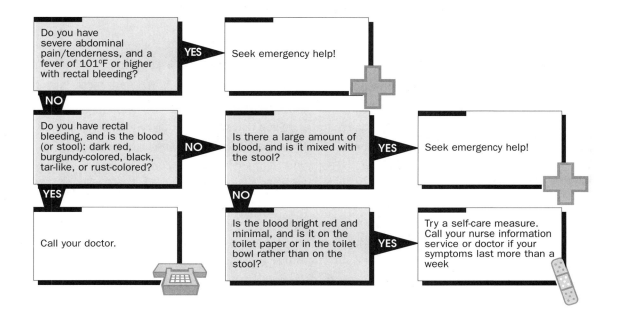

around the opening to the rectum, often in association with constipation and/or hemorrhoids. Fissures can usually be treated through self-care measures but occasionally require surgery.

Infectious diarrhea. You have sudden diarrhea, nausea and vomiting, headache, abdominal cramps, low-grade fever, and feel tired. Diarrhea may be caused by bacteria in contaminated food.

Colorectal cancer. You have dark, black, burgundy-colored, or rust-colored stools, or bright red rectal bleeding, along with one or more of the following: changes in bowel habits, diarrhea, constipation, bleeding between bowel movements, narrow stools, lower abdominal pain, bloating, cramps, excessive gas, loss of weight and appetite, or chronic fatigue. Colorectal cancer is very rarely the cause of rectal bleeding, but it's a consideration you should be aware of, especially if you're over the age of 50

and/or have a family history of colon or rectal cancer. If you have more than one of the above symptoms, and they do not go away, call your doctor.

Self-Care Measures
- If hemorrhoids are the cause, *see* page 167.

Prevention
- Since straining during bowel movements is frequently the cause of both hemorrhoids and anal fissures, try to avoid constipation by drinking plenty of water (6 to 8 glasses a day) and eating high-fiber foods (e.g., fruits, vegetables, beans, and whole-grain cereals).
- Exercise regularly.

RECTAL PAIN/ITCH

The Problem

You have pain and/or itching in your rectal area.

Causes of Rectal Pain and Itch

Poor hygiene. You have itching, but no pain or bleeding, in your rectal area. If the anal area is not cleansed adequately after a bowel movement, bits of stool can cling to the skin and cause irritation and itching.

Pinworms. You have anal itching that worsens at night, when you first go to bed, along with irritability and restless sleep. Pinworms generally infect young children, but other family members can become infected, too. You can determine whether this is the cause of the itching by getting a specimen: Wrap a piece of clear Scotch tape (sticky side out) around a flat, small object (e.g., a tongue depressor). Spread the buttocks, and press the tape firmly over the anal opening for a couple of minutes. Seal the sample in a plastic bag, and call your nurse information service or doctor.

Muscle spasm. You have a sharp, stabbing pain in your rectum that awakens you from a sound sleep, but may occur at any time. This condition is called proctalgia fugax and is most common among teenagers. It is believed to be caused by an intense spasm of the muscles near the rectum. It is not serious, and it usually disappears on its own.

Fungal infection. You have rectal itching; you may also be extremely hungry and thirsty, and you may notice that you are urinating more than usual. Anal itching can be caused by a fungal infection, usually *Candida* (i.e., yeast).

Self-Care Measures

- Cleanse the area gently (showering is best) in the morning, evening, and after each bowel movement. Rinse thoroughly. Do not use feminine hygiene deodorant sprays or powders.

Other Causes

Hemorrhoids (*see* page 164)
Contact dermatitis (*see* page 178)
Anal warts (*see* page 212)
Anal fissure (*see* page 164)
Proctitis
Sexually transmitted disease
 (*see* page 202)

Treating Your Child

- See *Self-Care Measures* and *Prevention* listed here.

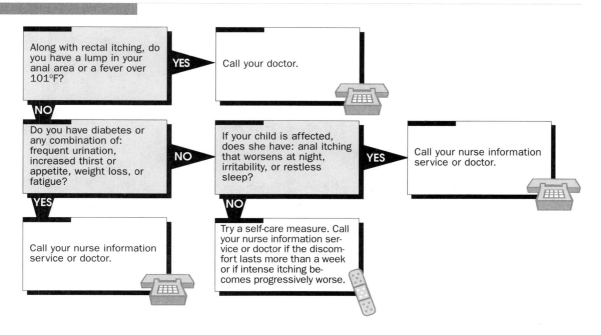

- To absorb any discharge and prevent skin irritation, place a cotton pad between your buttocks, up against the anal opening. Replace the pad as necessary.
- Wear cotton undergarments.
- Avoid eating citrus fruits (e.g., oranges, grapefruit, etc.) and spicy foods (e.g., curry or hot peppers).
- Limit yourself to 1 or 2 cups of coffee a day. Coffee beans contain oils that can't be digested, and they may irritate the skin around the anal area when they are excreted.
- Use plain, white, 2-ply toilet paper. Perfumes and dyes can be irritating to the skin and may cause allergic reactions.
- If hemorrhoids are the cause:
  - Take a sitz bath (available at drugstores) twice daily, for 15 to 30 minutes at a time.
  - Use soft toilet paper, preferably moistened with water, to clean yourself after bowel movements, and dry thoroughly afterward. Pat, don't rub. Disposable moist pads containing cleansing solutions are available over the counter and may be soothing.
  - Call your advice nurse before using over-the-counter creams or ointments designed to treat hemorrhoids.
  - If you have external, protruding hemorrhoids, tuck them back in with your finger after each bowel movement to avoid abrasion and irritation.

Prevention

- Keep the anal area clean and dry.
- Don't strain during bowel movements.

SCRAPE/ABRASION

The Problem

You have a shallow injury in which the top layers of your skin have been scraped off.

Important Information About Scrapes and Abrasions

In a scrape or abrasion, one or several layers of skin have been rubbed off by contact with something sharp or rough. Children, who fall more than adults and are more likely to engage in rough play or sports activities, are more prone to scrapes on knees, hands, and elbows. Even though they may cover a larger surface area and be more painful than cuts (*see* page 64), scrapes and abrasions tend to heal more quickly because they are superficial wounds.

Self-Care Measures

- Apply pressure with clean gauze or cloth to control bleeding.
- Wash the wound thoroughly with soap and warm water. If washing doesn't remove all of the dirt, you may have to soak the wound in clean, warm water.
- If the scrape has created a flap of skin, you can fold it carefully back in place if it is clean, but otherwise trim it away to minimize the risk of infection.
- If the abrasion is small or is not likely to bleed, leave it open.
- You can apply antibiotic creams or ointments (look for bacitracin as an ingredient) according to package directions, but don't use these products for more than 5 consecutive days. Cover any scrape that is still bleeding with a bandage, but take the bandage off as soon as the bleeding stops to speed healing. If healing has not started by then, call your nurse information service or doctor.

Treating Your Child

- Don't give aspirin to anyone under 19 years of age! It may cause a rare but serious problem called Reye's syndrome. Instead, use ibuprofen or acetaminophen (*see* page 27) for fever or pain.
- Make sure children wear helmets and other protective sports gear as appropriate.

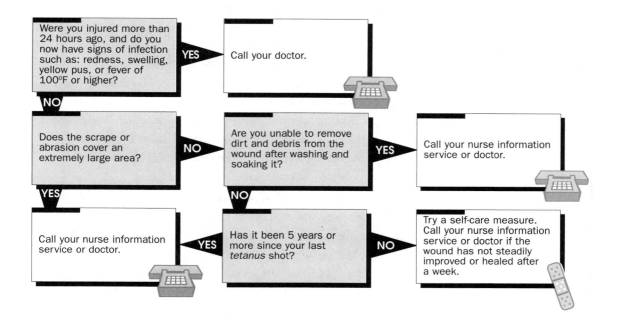

Were you injured more than 24 hours ago, and do you now have signs of infection such as: redness, swelling, yellow pus, or fever of 100°F or higher? **YES** → Call your doctor.

NO ↓

Does the scrape or abrasion cover an extremely large area? **NO** → Are you unable to remove dirt and debris from the wound after washing and soaking it? **YES** → Call your nurse information service or doctor.

YES ↓

Call your nurse information service or doctor. ← **YES** Has it been 5 years or more since your last *tetanus* shot? **NO** → Try a self-care measure. Call your nurse information service or doctor if the wound has not steadily improved or healed after a week.

- An ice pack may reduce swelling and ease discomfort. Use for 10 minutes on and 10 minutes off, until the pain subsides, generally within 48 to 72 hours.

- If necessary, use acetaminophen (*see* page 27) for pain relief.

- Do not use hydrogen peroxide or iodine on an open wound. They can hinder healing and may be painful.

- If your last tetanus shot was more than 5 years ago, you may need a booster. Call your nurse information service or doctor if you are uncertain about your immunization status.

- Remove the bandages and soak the wound 2 to 3 times a day for a few days and reapply the antibiotic cream or ointment and bandage.

- Observe the wound for signs of infection (e.g., redness, swelling, pus, and/or fever).

Prevention

- Many scrapes and abrasions are sustained while engaging in sports, such as skating or bicycling. Wear appropriate protective gear.

SEXUAL PROBLEM, MEN

The Problem

You're having difficulty with either sexual desire or performance.

Causes of Sexual Problems in Men

Other Causes

Peyronie's disease
Lack of orgasm
Delayed ejaculation
Painful intercourse

Impotence. You are unable to achieve or maintain an erection sufficient to have intercourse. Impotence, or erectile dysfunction, is an extremely common problem in men. It is important to realize that an occasional episode of impotence happens to nearly all men, is perfectly normal, and is nothing to be concerned about. If it becomes a persistent occurrence, however, it can be damaging to self-esteem and personal relationships. Fortunately, impotence is a very treatable problem.

Although impotence was once believed to be mainly psychologically caused, nearly half of impotence cases are now understood to have physical causes. (If you occasionally wake up with an erection, then your problem probably doesn't have a physical cause.) Possible psychological causes include depression (*see* page 238), lack of sexual desire, nervousness, fatigue, or so-called performance anxiety (the concern, after one episode of impotence, that the situation will occur again and again). Potential physical causes include, among others, diabetes (*see* page 240), heart disease (*see* page 236), hormone disorders, inflammation of the prostate gland (*see* page 254), excessive alcohol or other drug use, and side effects of prescription medications. Many cases of impotence clear up on their own.

Premature ejaculation. You reach orgasm and ejaculate following very brief stimulation and before you are able to satisfy your partner. This is one of the most common of all sexual problems in men, and it is particularly common in young men and/or those who are newly involved in a relationship. The causes are almost always of a psychological nature, usually the excitement and anxiety associated with initial sexual encounters.

Loss of sexual desire. You're not interested in sex anymore, and you seldom think about it. It's important to realize that loss of interest in sex affects everyone from time to time; you should consider it a problem only if it becomes a long-term condition and if you and/or your partner are dissatisfied as a result. Loss of desire may have several underlying causes. Depression (*see* page 238), fatigue, stress, pain, loss of interest, or unresolved conflict in a relationship may diminish your interest; however, a physical cause—for example, a drop in the male hormone testosterone—is another possibility.

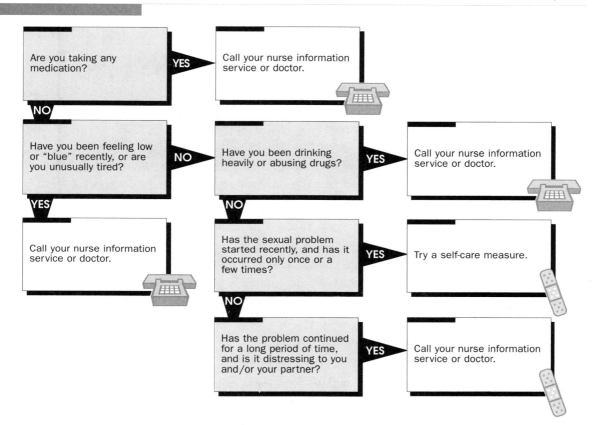

Self-Care Measures

- Books and videotapes about sex and sexual functioning are widely available and very useful.
- Relationship problems are at the root of many sexual difficulties, and open communication can make a tremendous difference.
- The "squeeze" technique, in which the woman squeezes her partner's penis just below the glans (i.e., head of the penis) between her thumb and forefinger when he signals that he is about to ejaculate, can help men who suffer from premature ejaculation gain greater control. Stopping stimulation and shifting positions before ejaculation can also restore control.
- Delayed ejaculation or inability to ejaculate may be caused by a drug (e.g., one of the newer antidepressants known as selective serotonin reuptake inhibitors [SSRIs]).
- If anxiety is the cause, sensate-focus exercises may help (*see* page 173).

Prevention

- Maintaining open, honest communication with your partner may help to prevent sexual problems from happening in the first place. Try to resolve your conflicts. Don't be hesitant about discussing any concerns you have about your sexual relationship.
- If you drink alcohol, have no more than 1 or 2 drinks a day.
- Don't use illicit drugs.
- Try to avoid overwork and fatigue.

SEXUAL PROBLEM, WOMEN

The Problem

You're having difficulty with either sexual desire or performance.

Causes of Sexual Problems in Women

Other Causes

Medication side effect

Vaginal dryness. Lack of vaginal lubrication can cause painful intercourse; this condition can result from insufficient foreplay for arousal, or it can occur when the body's estrogen production decreases after a menstrual period or at menopause. You may also notice vaginal dryness when using a decongestant cold medication.

Loss of sexual desire. You're simply not interested in sex; you may even find sex repulsive. It's important to recognize that all women go through periods when they don't desire sex; that's perfectly normal. It's reasonable to consider the situation a problem when it lasts a long time and when it causes relationship difficulties. Several medical conditions can cause diminished sexual interest and desire in women, but anger, relationship conflict, depression (*see* page 238), stress, alcohol, and fatigue are the most common causes.

Orgasmic dysfunction. You are not able to reach orgasm (climax) during sexual activity. Some women never reach orgasm during sexual activity with a partner and yet have pleasurable sexual experiences; others attain orgasm only some of the time or with certain kinds of stimulation; and still others reach orgasm every time they have intercourse. Causes can be physical, psychological, or both. Painful intercourse (see below) is one common physical cause, while psychological causes can include depression (*see* page 238), anger, or other feelings that affect the ability to focus on pleasurable sensations. Simple lack of knowledge about the anatomy and physiology of sexual response can be a cause. Some medications such as the newer antidepressants (called selective serotonin reuptake inhibitors, or SSRIs) can cause orgasm difficulty as a side effect. Self-care measures may help, but treatment is also an option.

Painful intercourse. You have discomfort or even extreme pain upon vaginal penetration. Painful intercourse, or dyspareunia, can be caused by several medical conditions, including vaginal irritation, infection (e.g., genital herpes [*see* page 42]), candidiasis (i.e., yeast infection [*see* page 208]), pelvic inflammatory disease [*see* page 208], growths, and endometriosis.

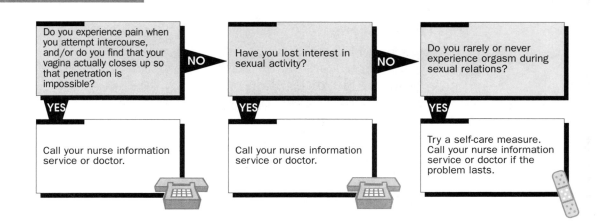

Vaginismus. You experience muscle spasms of the vagina when you attempt intercourse, and penetration becomes impossible. Vaginismus is an involuntary spasm of the muscles of the outer third of the vagina. Involuntary is the key word here; both the woman and her partner need to understand that this is not deliberate or willfully caused. The condition may be physical in origin, psychological, or both, but making the distinction requires a physical examination by a doctor.

Self-Care Measures

- You can remedy many sexual problems by using self-care measures. If these measures aren't effective after 6 months, however, call your nurse information service or doctor and ask about counseling.
  - You can improve vaginal dryness by using an over-the-counter, water-soluble lubricant (some lubricants can break down the latex in condoms, making them less effective; check with your pharmacist).
  - Many sexual difficulties arise out of anxiety in one or both partners. You and your partner may wish to try caressing each other without intercourse, using sensate-focus exercises. Touching in this way can be relaxing and can help to heighten both interest and arousal.
  - Some sexual difficulties are the result of a lack of knowledge. Take advantage of the many books and videotapes that have been designed to educate women about sexuality. Also, consider self-stimulation as a way of learning what is pleasurable to you.
  - A history of sexual abuse or rape can continue to haunt survivors long after the crisis has passed. If you are a survivor of abuse or rape, make sure you've gotten the professional help you need to work through the event to the greatest extent possible.

Prevention

- Avoid use of illicit drugs and excessive use of alcohol. These substances can affect sexual interest and responsiveness.
- Resolve relationship problems. Communicate openly, honestly, and frequently with your partner.

SHOULDER PAIN

The Problem
Your shoulder hurts.

Causes of Shoulder Pain

Bursitis. Your shoulder is tender and painful to the touch, perhaps even swollen. The twinges can become quite severe in a few hours, making it difficult to lift your arm. Bursitis is an inflammation of the bursae, which are fluid-filled sacs around joints that limit friction and make movement easier.

Tendinitis. You have muscle spasms and feel pain. Tendinitis is inflammation of a tendon, which connects muscle to bone.

Frozen shoulder. The shoulder may be painful or inflamed for no apparent reason or from overuse or abuse of the shoulder. If you try to avoid the pain by not moving the arm, the tissues will get stiff and the shoulder will become "frozen."

Other Causes

Sprain or strain (*see* page 182)
Shoulder *fracture*
Shoulder *dislocation*
Osteoarthritis (*see* page 224)
Rotator cuff tear
Gout (*see* page 108)
Pseudogout
Pneumonia
Ectopic pregnancy (*see* page 206)
Cholecystitis

Self-Care Measures

• In treating bursitis, your goal is first to rest your shoulder, then gradually exercise it to regain strength and range of motion. Try to avoid using your affected shoulder and arm for at least 1 to 4 days. To ease the pain, apply an ice pack or bag of frozen peas to the shoulder for 30 minutes, then off for 15; repeat this procedure for several hours. Then, gently perform normal range-of-motion movements several times a day to restore mobility (*see* figures). For strength, use hand weights during range-of-motion exercises.

• For tendinitis, try the RICE remedy: rest, ice, compression, elevation. Rest your shoulder for a day or so; you can resume activity gradually as you find that you're able to tolerate it. During

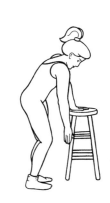
Rest your left hand on a flat surface at waist height. Drop your right hand down towards the floor.

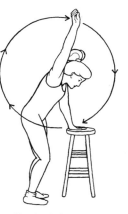
Slowly circle your arm forward and then backward. Repeat with the left arm.

Treating Your Child
• See *Self-Care Measures* and *Prevention* listed here.

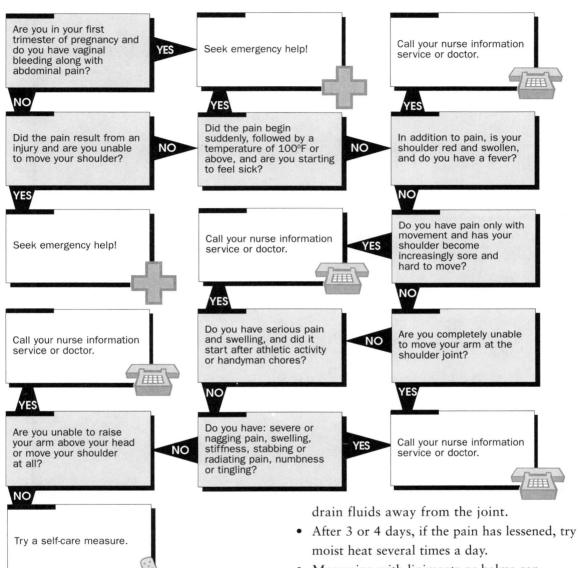

Are you in your first trimester of pregnancy and do you have vaginal bleeding along with abdominal pain?

YES → **Seek emergency help!**

NO ↓

YES → **Call your nurse information service or doctor.**

Did the pain result from an injury and are you unable to move your shoulder?

NO → **Did the pain begin suddenly, followed by a temperature of 100°F or above, and are you starting to feel sick?**

NO → **In addition to pain, is your shoulder red and swollen, and do you have a fever?**

YES ↓

Seek emergency help!

YES ↓ **Call your nurse information service or doctor.**

YES → **Do you have pain only with movement and has your shoulder become increasingly sore and hard to move?**

NO ↓

YES ↓ **Do you have serious pain and swelling, and did it start after athletic activity or handyman chores?**

NO → **Are you completely unable to move your arm at the shoulder joint?**

Call your nurse information service or doctor.

YES ↑

Are you unable to raise your arm above your head or move your shoulder at all?

NO → **Do you have: severe or nagging pain, swelling, stiffness, stabbing or radiating pain, numbness or tingling?**

YES → **Call your nurse information service or doctor.**

YES ↓ (from "Do you have serious pain..." NO)

NO ↓

Try a self-care measure.

the rest period, apply ice several times a day, 10 minutes on and 10 minutes off. Compress your shoulder by wrapping it snugly, but not tightly, with an elastic bandage. And finally, lie down, keeping your shoulder elevated to

drain fluids away from the joint.

- After 3 or 4 days, if the pain has lessened, try moist heat several times a day.
- Massaging with liniments or balms can increase blood flow and relax the muscles to help promote healing.

Prevention

- Avoid repetitive shoulder movement; vary your activities.

SINUS PAIN

The Problem

You've recently had a cold, and now you have severe nasal congestion with greenish-yellow mucus. You also have a feeling of pressure in your head, a headache that's at its worst when you wake up in the morning and when you bend forward, and/or pain over your cheeks. You may have a fever.

Other Causes

Allergic rhinitis (*see* page 256)
Acute sinusitis (*see* page 256)
Chronic sinusitis (*see* page 256)
Polyp
Cyst
Tumor
Foreign body (*see* page 153)
Wegener's granulomatosis

Causes of Sinus Pain

Common cold. Your nose is congested and/or running with clear to whitish mucus. You may be sneezing and coughing and have mild body aches and a low-grade fever. A cold is sometimes accompanied by mild sinus pain, but if your pain is moderate to severe, it's more likely that your cold (which is a viral infection) has progressed to sinusitis (which may be caused by bacteria). Colds are best treated with self-care measures.

Self-Care Measures

If your sinus pain is caused by a bacteria-related infection, you may need antibiotics. But you should use the following self-care measures either before or in addition to antibiotic treatment:

Treating Your Child

- Don't give aspirin to anyone under 19 years of age! It may cause a rare but serious problem called Reye's syndrome. Instead, use ibuprofen or acetaminophen (*see* page 27) for fever or pain.
- Children can also develop sinusitis, especially if they have allergies. When your child gets a cold, use a cool-mist vaporizer in her bedroom at night to help keep nasal secretions loose and draining.
- Over-the-counter oral decongestants may help, but use the ones made especially for children.
- If your child has a persistent nighttime cough that lasts longer than 2 weeks and a thick yellow or green nasal discharge, she may have a sinus infection.

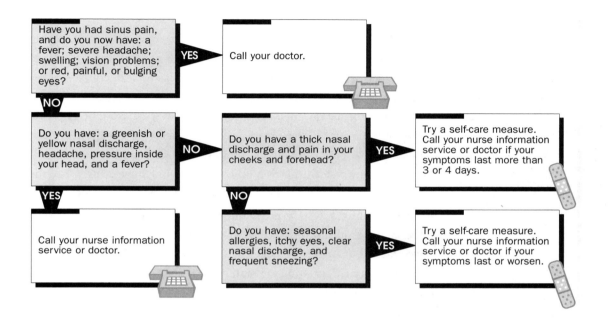

- Breathe moist, steamy air to help your sinuses drain. Take a hot shower twice a day. Buy a nasal steamer, or make your own by boiling a pot of water, removing it from the stove, draping a towel over your head and the pot, and inhaling the steam for 15 minutes, 3 times a day. Keep your head at least 18 inches from the water to avoid burning yourself.
- To help your sinuses drain during the night, elevate the head of your bed. You can do this by placing 6-inch wooden blocks under the legs of your headboard or by sleeping on a foam-rubber wedge.
- Over-the-counter oral or nasal decongestants can help, but don't use nasal decongestant sprays for more than 3 days. Doing so can cause a rebound effect that will make your congestion even worse.

- If a common cold is the cause, use aspirin, acetaminophen, or ibuprofen (*see* page 27) to reduce fever and muscle aches. Drink 6 to 8 glasses of fluid a day and get plenty of rest.

Prevention
- Allergies often set the stage for sinus infections, so either avoid exposure to anything you're allergic to or treat the underlying allergy with medications such as antihistamines, prescription nasal sprays, or desensitization shots.
- Avoid exposure to cigarette smoke; it is a severe sinus irritant.
- Drink plenty of water to keep nasal secretions loose.

SKIN, ITCHY/DRY

The Problem

Your skin is dry, itchy, and possibly cracked or irritated.

Causes of Itchy or Dry Skin

Other Causes

Hives (*see* page 124)
Scabies (*see* page 132)
Medication *allergy*
Parasite ("swimmer's itch")
Bug bite or sting (*see* page 184)
Ringworm (*see* page 106)
Athlete's foot (*see* page 98)
Poison ivy, oak, or sumac
Liver disease
Kidney disease
Blood disorder

Contact dermatitis. Your skin itches where it has been in contact with a new piece of jewelry or clothing, or you've recently switched detergents, skin creams, or deodorants; had your hair permed or dyed; or eaten some food or started a new medication to which you're allergic. You may also have a rash. When you scratch the rash, it may leave narrow, raised red lines exactly matching the track of your fingernails. Once the allergen is removed, the symptoms should fade.

Pruritis ("winter itch"). Your skin itches, probably on your lower legs, upper arms, flanks, or thighs. There may be no visible cause, or you may have cracked or irritated patches of skin. There's not enough humidity in your environment, or you may simply have dry skin because you are older. Self-care measures should control it.

Pityriasis rosea. You have one oval, itchy, scaly patch on your chest or back and similar, smaller patches on your upper arms, trunk, or thighs. This skin condition may last for 3 weeks to 3 months and then disappear without treatment; however, you may require medication to relieve the itch.

Self-Care Measures

- Avoid skin irritants.
- Limit baths and use warm, not hot, water when bathing. Use oil-based soaps sparingly; use lubricants without alcohol right after bathing, and pat, not rub, dry; and try over-the-counter moisturizing creams or lotions.
- Increase the humidity in your home, especially in the bedroom. Use

Treating Your Child

- See *Self-Care Measures* and *Prevention* listed here.

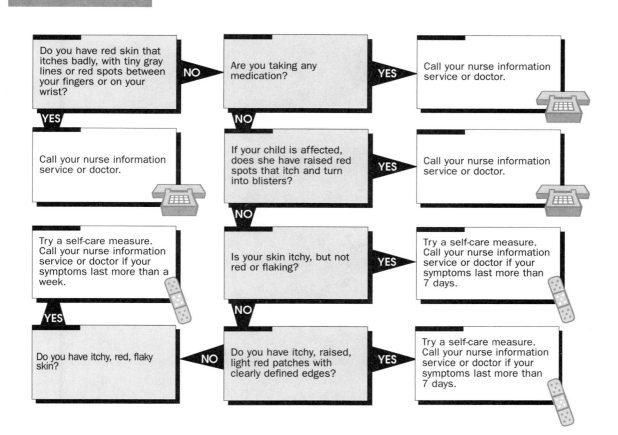

a humidifier or put a saucepan filled with water on top of the radiators.

- Take oatmeal baths or starch-and-soda baths: Tie a handful of regular oatmeal in a cheesecloth or cotton cloth, boil in water, and then sponge yourself with the ball (once it has cooled down enough to touch safely) in a lukewarm tub. Or soak in a lukewarm tub into which you have stirred 8 ounces of baking soda and 16 ounces of laundry starch. Do not use soap.

- Medications for itching have limited effects: Hydrocortisone creams (*see* page 28) may help

with the itch of contact dermatitis or eczema, but should not be used for prolonged periods unless your doctor recommends it. Use lanolin-containing creams cautiously; lanolin comes from sheep, and many people are allergic to sheep-related products.

Prevention

- Avoid excessively dry conditions.
- Identify and avoid allergens and irritants.

SPLINTER

The Problem
You have a sliver of wood or some other material stuck under your skin.

Important Information About Splinters
Unless they are very large, or very deep under a fingernail or toenail, nearly all splinters can be treated with self-care measures. The primary concern is infection, which is easily avoided by keeping the area clean.

Self-Care Measures
- Do not attempt to remove any large or deeply embedded splinter.
- If the splinter is made of wood, do not get the area wet. Water will cause the splinter to swell and make it more difficult to remove.
- Small splinters can be removed with a sterile pair of tweezers and a sharp needle. Wash your hands and sterilize the tweezers and needle by boiling them in water, soaking them in rubbing alcohol, or holding them over an open flame; cool before using. Try to grab the splinter with the tweezers. If you do not succeed, attempt to lift the splinter with the tip of the needle. Do not persistently poke with the needle, especially if the area becomes red and painful or if bleeding starts.
- After removing the splinter, wash the area thoroughly with soap and warm water, and use an antibiotic cream or ointment (look for bacitracin as an ingredient) and an adhesive bandage. Look for signs of infection during the next few days (e.g., redness, swelling, pus, and/or fever). Soak the affected area 3 to 4 times a day in warm, soapy water and apply the antibiotic cream or ointment and

Treating Your Child
- See *Self-Care Measures* and *Prevention* listed here.

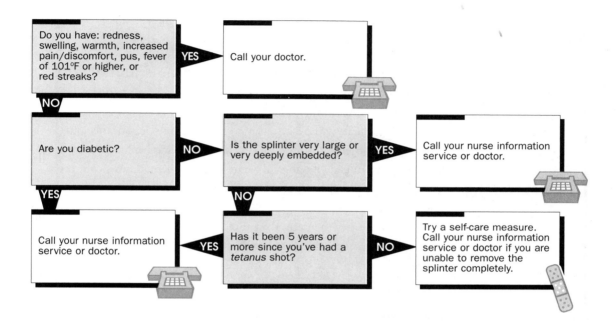

bandage for the next 4 or 5 days. Do not use bacitracin for more than 5 consecutive days. If healing has not started by then, call your nurse information service or doctor.

- If the splinter is very small, you may wait for it to come out on its own. Keep the area very clean to avoid infection.

Prevention

- Wear shoes or slippers when walking on wood floors or decks, and advise your children to do the same.
- Do not rub wood surfaces against the grain.
- Vacuum clean your floor or rug immediately, if you break an object made of glass or china.

SPRAIN/STRAIN

The Problem

You have injured one of your joints by sharply twisting it or by overusing it. You now have pain or tenderness in the area of the injury, and possibly swelling, redness, or bruising. You may also have difficulty moving the injured area.

Important Information About Sprains and Strains

Sprains and strains are injuries to the tissues that connect the bones of a joint and provide stability when the joint moves. A sprain is a stretched and torn ligament, while a strain is a stretched muscle. Sprains and strains occur when a trauma, such as a sudden twist or stretch, causes a joint to move outside its normal range of movement. They occur most often in the ankles, knees, and fingers, although any joint is susceptible. Sprains and strains vary in severity from minor to requiring surgery. In general, the greater the pain, the more serious the injury. Usually, self-care is all you need. An injured joint can usually bear weight within 24 hours and will be fully healed within 2 weeks.

Self-Care Measures

- Stop what you're doing the minute you feel pain. Try the RICE remedy: rest, ice, compression, and elevation. Rest the affected area for a day or so; you can resume activity gradually as you find that you're able to tolerate it. During the rest period, apply ice several times a day, 10 minutes on and 10 minutes off. Compress the area by wrapping it snugly, but not tightly, with an elastic bandage. And finally, keep the area elevated to drain fluids away from the joint.
- If you sprained a finger joint, remove any rings on the finger

Treating Your Child

- Don't give aspirin to anyone under 19 years of age! It may cause a rare but serious problem called Reye's syndrome. Instead, use ibuprofen or acetaminophen (see page 27) for fever or pain.

- Children may not be able to express feelings of pain, so observe very active children for signs of sprains and strains. If they suddenly stop their activity, begin to limp, or favor one side of their body over another, it may be a sign that they have an injury that requires medical attention.

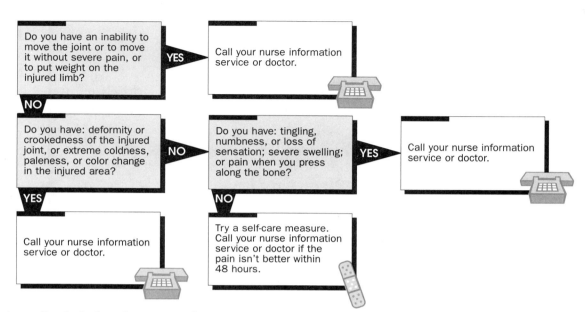

Do you have an inability to move the joint or to move it without severe pain, or to put weight on the injured limb?

YES → Call your nurse information service or doctor.

NO

Do you have: deformity or crookedness of the injured joint, or extreme coldness, paleness, or color change in the injured area?

NO → Do you have: tingling, numbness, or loss of sensation; severe swelling; or pain when you press along the bone?

YES → Call your nurse information service or doctor.

YES → Call your nurse information service or doctor.

NO → Try a self-care measure. Call your nurse information service or doctor if the pain isn't better within 48 hours.

immediately, before the joint swells.

- Take an over-the-counter pain reliever, such as aspirin or ibuprofen (*see* page 27), to relieve pain and swelling.

Prevention

- Many sprains and strains occur as a result of accidents in the home, so check your household for conditions that could lead to accidents:
  - Put handrails on stairways.
  - Use rubber mats in bathtubs and showers.
  - Make sure there are light switches near doors and steps.
  - Don't leave shoes, toys, tools, or other objects where people can trip over them.
- Sports injuries are another major cause of sprains and strains, so take these preventative measures:
  - Warm up with slow, easy stretches before starting any strenuous physical activity, and cool down for about 5 minutes following hard exercise (*see* figures).

- Don't overdo it. Pain is your body's way of telling you to ease up, so if your muscles or joints start to hurt, stop what you're doing.

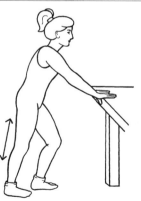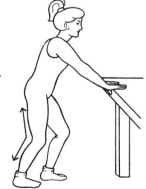

Stand with your hands on a flat surface at waist height. Step back with your right foot. Keep your right leg straight and bend your left leg, so that your weight is on your right foot. Feel the muscles stretch in the back of your right leg.

Bend your right knee, still keeping your weight off the left foot. Feel the muscles stretch in the front of your right leg. Repeat both stretches with your left leg.

STING/BITE, BUG

The Problem

You have a red lump or area on your skin that may itch or be swollen or painful. You may not be aware of having been bitten or stung.

Important Information About Stings and Bug Bites

Although they may be painful or cause terrible itching, bug bites or stings are rarely serious, except for bites by ticks, black widow spiders, brown recluse spiders, and scorpions. However, if you have an *allergic* reaction to the bite or sting, you may have more serious symptoms.

Bee sting. A bee has injected venom into your skin—that's the sting. The skin irritation and discomfort (including a small bump) should disappear after several days. However, you may have an allergic reaction to a bee sting. The symptoms include nausea and vomiting, difficulty breathing, and swelling around the eyes, lips, tongue, or throat; unconsciousness may also occur.

Black widow spider bite. The female black widow spider (so-called because it often eats its mate) has a glossy black body with a reddish hourglass mark on its belly. Its poisonous bite may be painless, but within hours you may experience cramping and a severe tightening of the muscles in the abdomen, nausea, convulsions, trouble breathing, perspiring, and vomiting.

Brown recluse, or "fiddleback," spider bite. You have a blue or purple mottled spot with a white ring around it, surrounded by a larger red ring. You were bitten by a brown spider somewhat smaller than a black widow

Treating Your Child

- Don't give aspirin to anyone under 19 years of age! It may cause a rare but serious problem called Reye's syndrome. Instead, use ibuprofen or acetaminophen (*see* page 27) for fever or pain.
- Poisonous spider bites are far more dangerous for children than adults; put ice or a cold compress on the bite, and seek emergency help!

- Most bites are not poisonous. Use the same self-care remedies as you would for adults. Commonly redness and swelling may develop a day later. If the area is itchy, this is simply a local reaction to a bite and cold packs are helpful. If the area is painful, there may be a secondary infection and you should call the doctor.

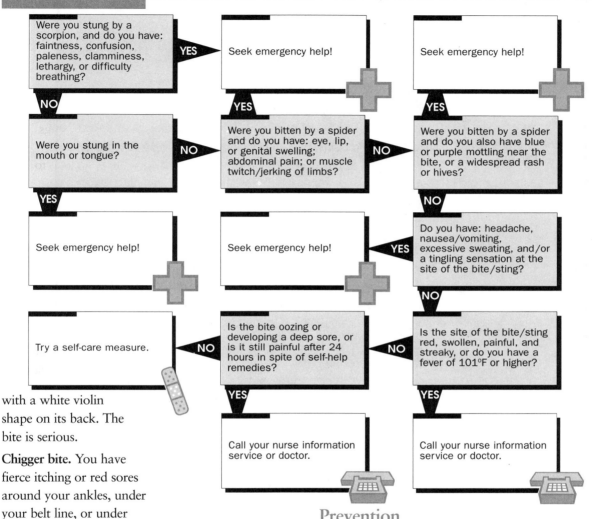

Were you stung by a scorpion, and do you have: faintness, confusion, paleness, clamminess, lethargy, or difficulty breathing?

YES → Seek emergency help!

NO

Were you stung in the mouth or tongue?

NO → Were you bitten by a spider and do you have: eye, lip, or genital swelling; abdominal pain; or muscle twitch/jerking of limbs?

YES → Seek emergency help!

NO → Were you bitten by a spider and do you also have blue or purple mottling near the bite, or a widespread rash or hives?

YES → Seek emergency help!

YES

Seek emergency help!

YES → Seek emergency help!

NO

Do you have: headache, nausea/vomiting, excessive sweating, and/or a tingling sensation at the site of the bite/sting?

YES → Seek emergency help!

NO

Try a self-care measure.

NO ← Is the bite oozing or developing a deep sore, or is it still painful after 24 hours in spite of self-help remedies?

NO ← Is the site of the bite/sting red, swollen, painful, and streaky, or do you have a fever of 101°F or higher?

YES

Call your nurse information service or doctor.

YES

Call your nurse information service or doctor.

with a white violin shape on its back. The bite is serious.

Chigger bite. You have fierce itching or red sores around your ankles, under your belt line, or under openings in your clothes. You've been in contact with grass or shrubs. You can see small red mites or red spots in the centers of the sores.

Self-Care Measures

- For all kinds of bites: Use ice or cold compresses immediately, even if the bite is serious and you've called for emergency help. Try an over-the-counter pain reliever.
- If itching is a problem, *see* page 178.
- Do not use kerosene, gasoline, or alcohol on ticks.

Prevention

- Avoid high grass, woods, bushes, and other places where you may come in contact with insects. Wear protective clothing. Use insect repellents containing DEET (diethyltoluamide). Do not use DEET on children under 2 years and be careful when applying insect repellents around the eyes.
- When around bees, avoid brightly colored clothes.
- Regularly inspect yourself, children, and pets for ticks.
- Avoid products with scents such as perfume, scented hair spray, and deodorant.

185

STOMACH PAIN/CRAMPING

The Problem

You have pain or cramping anywhere between your ribs and groin.

Causes of Stomach Pain

Irritable bowel syndrome. You have stomach pain, diarrhea, and constipation. The cause of irritable bowel syndrome is unknown, but stress, dairy products, and high-fat or gas-producing foods may make it worse. You can help avoid irritable bowel syndrome or lessen its symptoms by eating a low-fat, high-fiber diet, exercising moderately, and managing stress.

Female reproductive problem. You have severe stomach pain, and you are pregnant or might be. This is potentially serious, so seek emergency help! Recurrent pain other than ordinary menstrual cramps, just before or during menstruation, may mean *endometriosis*. Severe, one-sided pain in your lower abdomen with fever and occasionally a vaginal discharge could signal a sexually transmitted disease (*see* page 202).

Self-Care Measures

If you have severe or lasting pain, you should absolutely not rely on self-care measures, especially over-the-counter remedies and laxatives. Otherwise, try the following:

- For mild pains or pain caused by something you ate, try sipping water or sucking on crushed ice for a few hours. For the next 24 hours, drink water or clear fluids; avoid solid foods. Then slowly start trying

Other Causes

Gastroenteritis (*see* page 148)
Heartburn (*see* page 118)
Urinary tract infection
  (*see* page 94)
Diverticulitis
Peptic ulcer or gastritis
  (*see* page 252)
Kidney stone (*see* page 204)
Appendicitis
Abdominal injury
Duodenal *ulcer*
Peritonitis
Cholecystitis
Crohn's disease
Intestinal obstruction

Treating Your Child

- Don't give aspirin to anyone under 19 years of age! It may cause a rare but serious problem called Reye's syndrome. Instead, use ibuprofen or acetaminophen (*see* page 27) for fever or pain.
- If your child screams with pain at the slightest movement or touch or has any blood in his stool, seek emergency help!
- *Colic* is often the reason that infants between the age of 2 weeks and 3 to 4 months cry for a long time without apparent reason, especially if they stop crying after the passage of gas or a bowel movement. Typically, babies with colic have excellent appetites. If your baby stops eating and seems to have abdominal pain, consult your nurse information service or doctor.

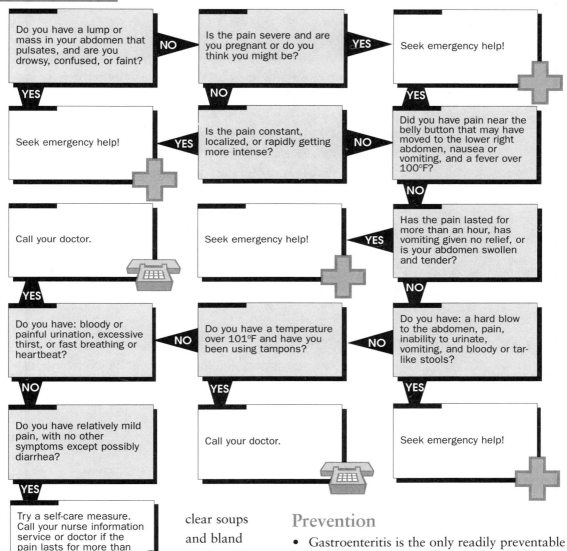

Do you have a lump or mass in your abdomen that pulsates, and are you drowsy, confused, or faint? — **NO** → Is the pain severe and are you pregnant or do you think you might be? — **YES** → Seek emergency help!

Do you have a lump or mass in your abdomen that pulsates, and are you drowsy, confused, or faint? — **YES** → Seek emergency help!

Is the pain severe and are you pregnant or do you think you might be? — **NO** → Is the pain constant, localized, or rapidly getting more intense? — **NO** → Did you have pain near the belly button that may have moved to the lower right abdomen, nausea or vomiting, and a fever over 100°F?

Is the pain constant, localized, or rapidly getting more intense? — **YES** → Seek emergency help!

Seek emergency help! → Call your doctor.

Did you have pain near the belly button that may have moved to the lower right abdomen, nausea or vomiting, and a fever over 100°F? — **NO** → Has the pain lasted for more than an hour, has vomiting given no relief, or is your abdomen swollen and tender?

Has the pain lasted for more than an hour, has vomiting given no relief, or is your abdomen swollen and tender? — **YES** → Seek emergency help!

Call your doctor. — **YES** → Do you have: bloody or painful urination, excessive thirst, or fast breathing or heartbeat?

Has the pain lasted for more than an hour, has vomiting given no relief, or is your abdomen swollen and tender? — **NO** → Do you have: a hard blow to the abdomen, pain, inability to urinate, vomiting, and bloody or tar-like stools?

Do you have: bloody or painful urination, excessive thirst, or fast breathing or heartbeat? — **NO** → Do you have a temperature over 101°F and have you been using tampons? — **NO** → Do you have: a hard blow to the abdomen, pain, inability to urinate, vomiting, and bloody or tar-like stools?

Do you have a temperature over 101°F and have you been using tampons? — **YES** → Call your doctor.

Do you have: a hard blow to the abdomen, pain, inability to urinate, vomiting, and bloody or tar-like stools? — **YES** → Seek emergency help!

Do you have: bloody or painful urination, excessive thirst, or fast breathing or heartbeat? — **NO** → Do you have relatively mild pain, with no other symptoms except possibly diarrhea?

Do you have relatively mild pain, with no other symptoms except possibly diarrhea? — **YES** → Try a self-care measure. Call your nurse information service or doctor if the pain lasts for more than 24 hours.

clear soups and bland foods such as toast and oatmeal. Don't restrain the passage of gas or bowel movements; this often brings relief.

- Rest. Take acetaminophen (*see* page 27) for fever.
- If heartburn is the cause, *see* page 118.
- If diarrhea is the cause, *see* page 68.

Prevention

- Gastroenteritis is the only readily preventable cause of abdominal pain. Make sure meats, mayonnaise, shellfish (especially raw oysters), and poultry are properly refrigerated; never eat any of these foods if left unrefrigerated for more than 2 hours.
- Avoid irritation from repeated long-term use of aspirin or nonsteroidal anti-inflammatory drugs (NSAIDs).
- Avoid excessive alcohol intake.

SUNBURN

The Problem

Your skin is red, slightly swollen, very painful, and possibly blistered, and you've just spent time in the sun. If your sunburn is extensive and severe, you may also have chills, fever, nausea, and vomiting.

Important Information About Sunburn

Sunburn is generally caused by too much exposure to *ultraviolet* (UV) light. The sun's UV rays are not screened out by thin clouds, so it's possible to get sunburned even on overcast days. Sand, snow, and water reflect the sun's rays, causing you to sunburn at a faster rate while at the beach or participating in snow or water sports. People with little melanin in their skin—those who are fair and have blue eyes and blond or red hair—are at greatest risk for sunburn. Certain medications, including sulfa-containing drugs, tetracyclines, amoxicillin, oral contraceptives, and some diuretics, can also increase your sensitivity to the sun.

Self-Care Measures

Use the following self-care measures to make yourself more comfortable while your skin heals. Be assured that the pain of a sunburn is at its worst 6 to 48 hours after sun exposure.

Treating Your Child

- Don't give aspirin to anyone under 19 years of age! It may cause a rare but serious problem called Reye's syndrome. Instead, use ibuprofen or acetaminophen (*see* page 27) for fever or pain.
- Children can play in the sun for hours unaware that they're getting sunburned. Therefore, be vigilant about your child's sun exposure, and insist that he wear a sunscreen, a hat, and protective clothing. However, don't use sunscreen on very young children; try to keep them out of the sun.
- The same self-care measures that work for adults will also work for children.

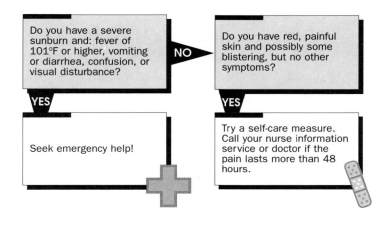

Do you have a severe sunburn and: fever of 101°F or higher, vomiting or diarrhea, confusion, or visual disturbance?

NO

Do you have red, painful skin and possibly some blistering, but no other symptoms?

YES

Seek emergency help!

YES

Try a self-care measure. Call your nurse information service or doctor if the pain lasts more than 48 hours.

- To reduce heat and pain, make cool compresses by dipping towels or strips of gauze in cool water and laying them on the burned areas.
- Take a cool soak in an oatmeal bath (preparations are available over the counter) or in a bath with baking soda (add half a cup of baking soda to a tub full of water).
- Avoid products containing benzocaine unless otherwise advised by your doctor. They may temporarily numb the skin, but they can be irritating and may actually delay healing by triggering an allergic reaction.
- Try an over-the-counter pain reliever, such as aspirin, acetaminophen, or ibuprofen (*see* page 27).
- Rest in a comfortable position in a cool, quiet room.
- Drink plenty of water to replace lost fluids.

Prevention

- You're far better off preventing sunburn than trying to treat it once it's occurred. In addition to causing severe pain and discomfort, sunburn can age your skin before its time and can place you at risk for skin cancer. Avoid the sun's rays between the hours of 11 a.m. and 3 p.m. If you must be outside during this time, wear a hat, protective clothing, and a sunblock (not a lotion designed for suntanning) with a sun protective factor (SPF) of 15 or more. Reapply after swimming or excessive sweating, and after prolonged exposure to the sun.

SWALLOWING DIFFICULTY

The Problem

You have discomfort or pain when swallowing, and you may have difficulty getting food to go down at all.

Causes of Swallowing Difficulty

Other Causes

Heartburn (*see* page 118)
Hiatal hernia (*see* page 118)
Ulcer
Cigarette smoking
Aortic *aneurysm*
Botulism
Goiter
Cancer
Parkinson's disease
Neuralgia
Tetanus
Thyroiditis
Wilson's disease
Anaphylaxis
Esophageal stricture

Infection. You're having trouble swallowing, and you also have a sore throat, a fever, and possibly other symptoms (e.g., a headache, fatigue, and loss of appetite). A viral or bacterial infection anywhere in the area of the upper respiratory tract can lead to difficulty swallowing; your other symptoms will vary depending on the location of the infection.

Foreign body. You're having trouble swallowing; your throat is sore; and you might have swallowed something small and sharp, like a fish bone.

Anxiety/stress. You swallow normally, but then you feel as though the food gets stuck and will not go down or as though you have a lump in your throat. This feeling can be a symptom of stress and anxiety. Increasing your fluid intake while eating may help. You may also wish to call your nurse information service or doctor and ask about stress management and relaxation techniques.

Self-Care Measures

Swallowing difficulties can often be treated with self-care measures.

- If anxiety/stress is the cause, using a relaxation technique may help. If you are hyperventilating, try breathing into a paper bag (*see* page 48).

Treating Your Child

- Throat infections and other infections of the upper respiratory tract are quite common in children, so if your child complains of difficulty swallowing, look for other symptoms of infection. If your child also has throat pain and a fever that doesn't subside after 2 days, call your nurse information service or doctor.
- Because of their small size, children can dehydrate much more quickly than adults.

Make sure that swallowing difficulty isn't interfering with your child's ability to take in enough fluids. Call your nurse information service or doctor if you note symptoms of dehydration (e.g., dry diaper for more than 3 hours or infrequent urination for more than 12 hours, no tears, dry mouth, sunken eyes, loss of skin elasticity, and unusual lethargy or irritability).

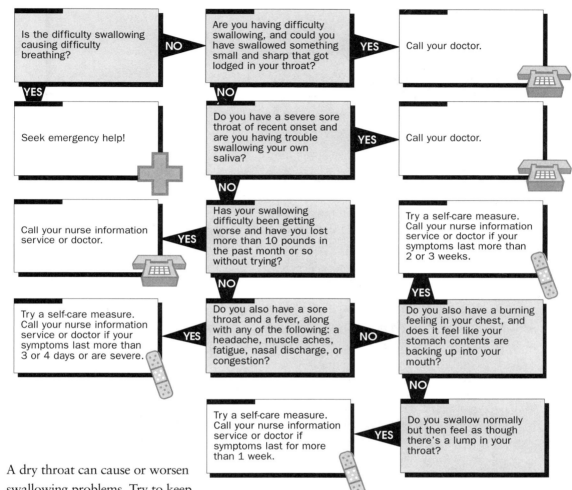

- A dry throat can cause or worsen swallowing problems. Try to keep yourself well hydrated, and make sure the air in your home isn't too dry. Drink plenty of liquid each day, and try a cool-mist vaporizer in your bedroom at night.

- If heartburn is causing your problem, there are many things you can do to relieve it. Losing weight almost always helps, as does eating smaller, frequent meals. Avoid coffee, alcohol, and smoking. Try an over-the-counter antacid, drink a glass of milk, or eat some bread to relieve the pain. Avoid bending over or lying down after a

meal, and try raising the head of your bed by about 4 inches to prevent stomach acid from backing up into your throat.

Prevention

- If your problem is caused by stress and anxiety, try learning some relaxation exercises. You'll find many good books, audiotapes, and videotapes on the subject at your local library or bookstore.

191

SWEATINESS

The Problem

You are perspiring excessively.

Causes of Sweatiness

Obesity. You are overweight, and you sweat a lot. Carrying around too many pounds puts a strain on your body, so that even everyday activities can cause excessive sweating. Losing weight will help significantly. For more information on obesity, *see* page 248.

Menopause. You are over 38 years old, and your periods have become irregular. You notice that you often become very warm quite suddenly and begin to sweat profusely. You may also have sweating episodes at night. These episodes, referred to as menopausal *hot flashes* and night sweats, are common and completely normal symptoms of menopause. Some women choose to tolerate them, while others try one of many treatments available. Discuss your symptoms with your doctor during your next appointment.

Hyperthyroidism. In addition to excessive sweating, you've also had unexplained weight loss, an increase in appetite, weakness or trembling, bulging of your eyes, and/or rapid heartbeat. This problem is not dangerous as long as it's treated promptly.

Other Causes

Heat and humidity
Physical exertion
Fever (*see* page 94)
Anxiety or stress
Puberty
Medication side effect
Alcohol use
Alcohol withdrawal
Aspirin use
Pneumonia
Infection
Heart disease (*see* page 236)
Liver disease

Self-Care Measures

Sweating is a natural mechanism for regulating body temperature. Some people naturally perspire a lot; if you're one of those people, there is probably nothing wrong. There are many things you can do, however, to diminish the problem and make yourself more comfortable.

- Dress in natural, light, loose-fitting fabrics, like cotton, that absorb perspiration and allow air to circulate. Avoid manufactured fibers like rayon, nylon, and polyester.

Treating Your Child

- If your child is a teenager who is complaining of sweatiness, let him know that the development of additional sweat glands during puberty causes an increase in perspiration that is particularly noticeable under the arms. Reassure him that this is perfectly normal and is no reason for embarrassment. Showering regularly and using an antiperspirant will reduce the wetness and prevent unpleasant body odor.

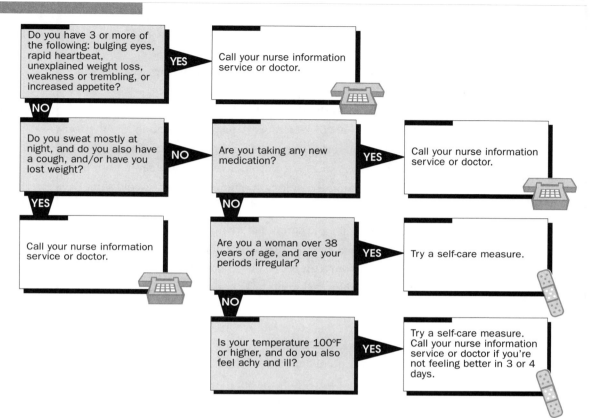

Do you have 3 or more of the following: bulging eyes, rapid heartbeat, unexplained weight loss, weakness or trembling, or increased appetite?

YES → Call your nurse information service or doctor.

NO ↓

Do you sweat mostly at night, and do you also have a cough, and/or have you lost weight?

NO → Are you taking any new medication?

YES → Call your nurse information service or doctor.

YES ↓

Call your nurse information service or doctor.

NO ↓

Are you a woman over 38 years of age, and are your periods irregular?

YES → Try a self-care measure.

NO ↓

Is your temperature 100°F or higher, and do you also feel achy and ill?

YES → Try a self-care measure. Call your nurse information service or doctor if you're not feeling better in 3 or 4 days.

- Use a deodorant that contains an antiperspirant (some offer only masking fragrances and do not contain an antiperspirant). Choose roll-on or stick antiperspirants; they provide more protection than sprays. Dry yourself thoroughly before applying your antiperspirant, as moisture will dilute its effectiveness. An antiperspirant may be applied to any area of your body that perspires excessively, including your feet, the palms of your hands, and your forehead.

- Soak the problem areas (e.g., the palms of your hands) in cool water for approximately 30 minutes. This may prevent sweating for up to 3 hours.

- Avoid hot, spicy food.

- Do not smoke, and if you drink alcohol, do so in moderation; both of these increase sweating.

- If your problem is severe, and none of the self-care measures are effective, you might try iontophoresis— a technique in which a weak electrical current is applied to particularly problematic areas. Iontophoresis constricts the sweat ducts and controls perspiration. A device for this purpose (called a drionic) is available without a prescription; or call your nurse information service or doctor and ask about having the procedure done in the doctor's office.

Prevention

- Shower at least once a day. This won't eliminate your perspiration problem, but it will help to ensure that the perspiration doesn't have an unpleasant odor.

THIRST, EXCESSIVE

The Problem

Your mouth is very dry; you may also have dry lips and dry skin.

Causes of Excessive Thirst

Other Causes

Dehydration
Medication side effect
Diabetes mellitus (*see* page 240)
Diabetes insipidus
Internal bleeding

Peritonitis. You have severe, steady pain in your abdomen that gets worse when you move or put pressure on the area. Your abdomen is rigid and swollen, or bloated. You have chills and fever, with profuse sweating, nausea and vomiting, weakness, and pale, cold skin. Bacteria, particularly those found within the intestine, can cause *peritonitis*.

Sunstroke or heat exhaustion. Following hours spent in strong sunlight or high heat, your temperature is 103°F or higher. You are not sweating, and your skin is dry, even under the armpits. You may be confused or cranky, feel faint, have muscle cramps, lose consciousness, or have a seizure.

Self-Care Measures

- Drink an adequate amount of fluids. Generally our bodies tell us when we need fluids by making us feel thirsty. Pay attention to your thirst, especially if you are perspiring heavily or when your daily intake of water should be more than the 6 to 8 glasses of water usually recommended.
- Drink water before, during, and after exercise. If you're involved in a particularly strenuous workout, drink sports drinks. They not only supply fluids, but they also replace electrolytes (i.e., minerals that

Treating Your Child

- Children often ignore thirst because they are easily distracted. When your child is vomiting, has diarrhea, or is playing outside in hot weather, make sure she drinks fluids frequently.
- Because of their small size, infants and young children can dehydrate much more quickly than adults. Be alert for the following signs of dehydration if your child is vomiting and/or has diarrhea, and seek emergency help if you observe them: dry diaper for more than 5 hours or small amounts of urine for more than 12 hours, unusual lethargy or irritability, lack of skin elasticity, and very little saliva or tears.

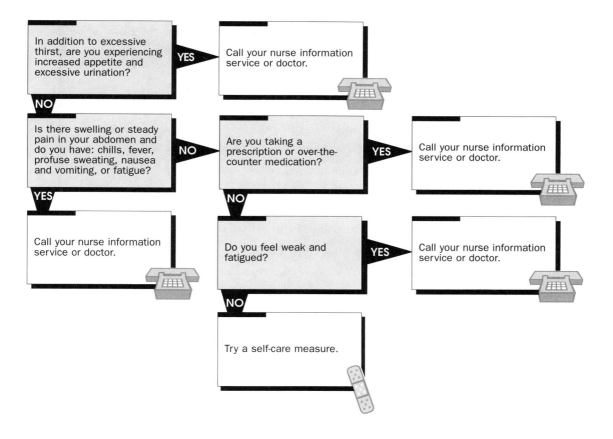

In addition to excessive thirst, are you experiencing increased appetite and excessive urination?

YES → Call your nurse information service or doctor.

NO

Is there swelling or steady pain in your abdomen and do you have: chills, fever, profuse sweating, nausea and vomiting, or fatigue?

NO → Are you taking a prescription or over-the-counter medication?

YES → Call your nurse information service or doctor.

YES → Call your nurse information service or doctor.

NO

Do you feel weak and fatigued?

YES → Call your nurse information service or doctor.

NO

Try a self-care measure.

are essential for the normal functioning of all cells in the body), which you lose when you perspire.

- If peritonitis is the cause, an over-the-counter analgesic may ease the pain.
- If you think you're dehydrated (i.e., you have severe thirst, infrequent urination or dark yellow urine, eyes that appear sunken, or inelastic skin) due to vomiting, suck on ice chips or frozen fruit bars. Sip clear fluid, such as clear soup, tea (no milk), water, or sports drinks; you can also try slightly flat ginger ale, cola, or ginger tea. As you begin to feel better, work your way up to juices, soups, gelatin, and applesauce.

Prevention

- Stay hydrated by drinking plenty of fluids. If you have a water-softening system in your home, consider buying bottled water for drinking. Softening water removes its calcium and magnesium and replaces them with sodium, which can make you thirsty.

THROAT PAIN

The Problem
Your throat hurts and is red. It may be painful to swallow.

Causes of Throat Pain

Other Causes

Allergy
Cigarette smoking
Head cold
Heartburn (*see* page 118)
Sinusitis (*see* page 256)
Epiglottitis
Influenza
Thyroiditis
Measles
Tonsillitis (*see* page 103)
Mononucleosis (*see* page 102)
Chronic fatigue syndrome

Pharyngitis. Your throat is inflamed and sore. You may have fever, swollen glands, and difficulty swallowing. The cause may be a virus or bacterium.

Strep throat. Strep throat is caused by a bacterium called streptococcus. It is more common in children than adults and is very contagious. It is usually associated with fever, pain with swallowing, swollen glands under the jaw, and white spots on the back of the throat. Strep throat is diagnosed with a lab test and treated with antibiotics to prevent complications, which can be serious.

Laryngitis. Your vocal cords are inflamed and swollen. You may be hoarse or lose your voice. The cause is usually a virus or allergy, or overuse of your voice. Laryngitis can usually be treated with self-care measures.

Mumps. The glands in front of and below your ears may be swollen; you may not be able to feel your jawbone. Other common signs are fever and vomiting. Mumps is caused by a virus.

Treating Your Child
- Don't give aspirin to anyone under 19 years of age! It may cause a rare but serious problem called Reye's syndrome. Instead, use ibuprofen or acetaminophen (*see* page 27) for fever or pain.
- If your child is having trouble swallowing, or is drooling more than usual, call your nurse information service or doctor.
- Almost all respiratory illnesses are spread through saliva, so avoid sharing eating utensils. Give hugs, not kisses. Wash your child's hands and your own frequently.
- While most respiratory illnesses last 7 to 10 days, some such as infectious mononucleosis or "mono" (*see* page 102) may cause throat pain for weeks.

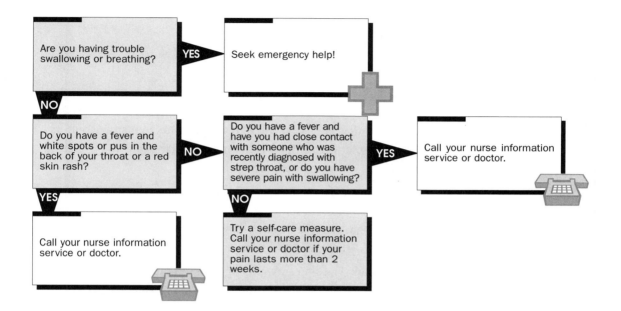

Self-Care Measures

- To relieve pain, take an over-the-counter pain medicine such as aspirin (*see* page 27). If the feeling in your throat makes you cough, try cough drops or hard candy. For runny nose, take a decongestant (with or without an antihistamine).

- To soothe your throat, try one or more of the following:
  - Suck on hard candy.
  - Drink plenty of fluids. Try soup, or tea with honey and/or lemon.
  - Gargle every few hours with salt water (1/4 teaspoon of salt in 8 ounces of warm water) or an over-the-counter mouthwash.

- If dry air is the cause, a humidifier or vaporizer—or even a pan of water on the radiator—will moisten the air and provide relief.

- If voice overuse (e.g., yelling, singing, or excessive speaking) is the cause, rest your voice.

- If smoking is the cause, try to cut down or stop smoking (*see* page 24).

Prevention

- Depending on the cause, there may be steps you can take to prevent recurrence of your throat pain. The key is to avoid the cause. For example, if you smoke, try to stop. If the air in your home or office is dry, keep it moist. If you are overusing your voice, try to stop. If heartburn is the cause, *see* page 118.

TOE PAIN

The Problem

You have soreness in one or more of your toes.

Causes of Toe Pain

Hammertoe. Your toe (probably the second one) is painful and bent, with an arched, clawlike appearance. Hammertoe can result from wearing shoes that are too small, but it also occurs in many people as they age. It also affects people with long-term diabetes who have nerve damage as a result of their condition.

Mallet toe. Your toe is painful, and it curls under at the tip. Like hammertoe, mallet toe is frequently caused by poorly fitting shoes; in this case, though, the shoes usually have high heels and pointy toes that squeeze the front of the foot.

Ingrown toenail. The skin surrounding your toenail is red, swollen, and painful; it may also be discharging greenish or yellowish fluid. An ingrown toenail occurs when the sharp end of a toenail grows into the skin of the toe (usually the big toe). It can result from poor-fitting shoes or from improper cutting of the toenails. Unless you are diabetic or have symptoms of infection (e.g., green or yellow discharge), self-care is usually all that this condition requires.

Other Causes

Bunion or *bunionette*
Osteoarthritis (*see* page 224)
Infection
Gout (*see* page 108)
Fracture
Frostbite
Poorly fitting shoes
Neuropathy

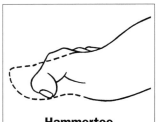

Hammertoe

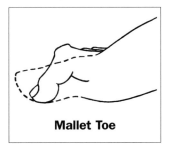

Mallet Toe

Self-Care Measures

- For hammertoe or mallet toe, try wearing sandals; often, simply eliminating the pressure that regular shoes place on the tops of crooked toes is enough to eliminate the discomfort. Try placing a crest pad—a tapered foam cushion available at medical-supply stores—under your toes to prevent them from curling under. If you are extremely uncomfortable, surgery may be necessary to correct the problem.

Treating Your Child

- See *Self-Care Measures* and *Prevention* listed here.

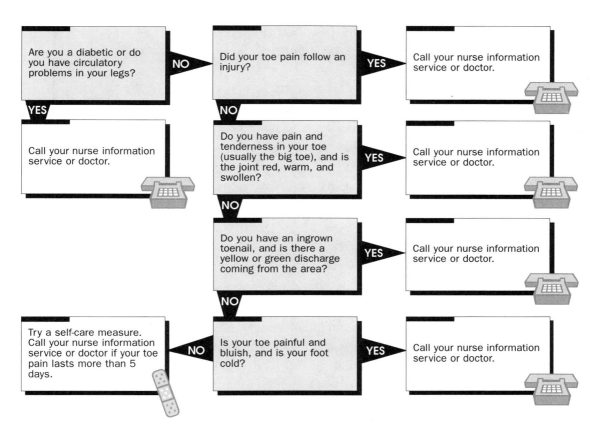

Are you a diabetic or do you have circulatory problems in your legs?

NO → **Did your toe pain follow an injury?** → YES → Call your nurse information service or doctor.

YES → Call your nurse information service or doctor.

NO ↓ **Do you have pain and tenderness in your toe (usually the big toe), and is the joint red, warm, and swollen?** → YES → Call your nurse information service or doctor.

NO ↓ **Do you have an ingrown toenail, and is there a yellow or green discharge coming from the area?** → YES → Call your nurse information service or doctor.

NO ↓

Try a self-care measure. Call your nurse information service or doctor if your toe pain lasts more than 5 days. ← NO ← **Is your toe painful and bluish, and is your foot cold?** → YES → Call your nurse information service or doctor.

- If you have an ingrown toenail, try soaking your foot in a basin of warm water, mixed with 2 tablespoons of table salt, for 15 to 20 minutes. Then, gently massage the skin away from the trapped nail. After the nail and skin have been separated, place a small piece of cotton or net tissue between the nail and the skin for a few days, until the nail grows out and the skin heals. (Note: Do not use this self-care measure if you are diabetic or have circulatory problems, or if the ingrown toenail is infected.)

Prevention

- Wear shoes that fit comfortably, such as low-heel shoes with square or rounded toes. Have a professional measure your feet from time to time; foot size can change.
- When cutting your toenails, be sure to cut them straight across. Use a pair of toenail clippers instead of small, rounded fingernail clippers; they'll make it easier to make a straight cut. Because toenails are thick, the best time to cut them is after bathing, when they're soft.

TOOTH PAIN

The Problem

You have pain—dull, throbbing, or sharp—in your tooth or teeth.

Causes of Toothache

Tooth decay. Your tooth throbs. The pain goes away but keeps coming back, triggered by both hot and cold food or liquids and by breathing cold air. You may have a deep cavity or filling or an injury to the tooth that has inflamed the nerve in the inner tooth pulp. The most common cause of tooth decay is excessive use of sugar coupled with poor dental hygiene. Sugar is a good medium for bacteria to produce acid, which attacks the protective enamel on your teeth, gets inside, and causes inflammation and pain.

Recent dental work. You just had a filling, and now your tooth hurts for a few seconds when you bite on it.

Gum disease. Your gums bleed easily, may be receding and are red-purple, swollen, and shiny, and your teeth are sensitive to hot and cold. You have bad breath. This is probably gingivitis, a disease that causes the gums to shrink away from the base of the teeth, leaving sensitive areas exposed to temperature shock.

Abscess. You have continuous pain, an uncomfortable "bite," a loose tooth, or a fever. You could have an abscess, which is the result of pus building up around a tooth with a cavity, an injury, or gum disease that creates a "pocket" near the base of the tooth.

Temporomandibular joint (TMJ) syndrome. Your jaw joint is inflamed/swollen, and you may have pain in your head, face, teeth, neck, and/or shoulders. Your ears may be ringing and you may hear clicking sounds when you open or shut your mouth. TMJ syndrome occurs when the muscles and ligaments around the jawbone are stretched too far or are out of alignment.

Other Causes

Cracked tooth or filling
Impacted tooth
Sinusitis (*see* page 256)
Neuralgia

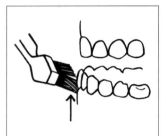

Start with the toothbrush on your gum and brush upward away from the gumline.

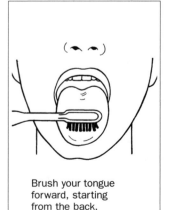

Brush your tongue forward, starting from the back.

Treating Your Child

- See *Self-Care Measures* and *Prevention* listed here.

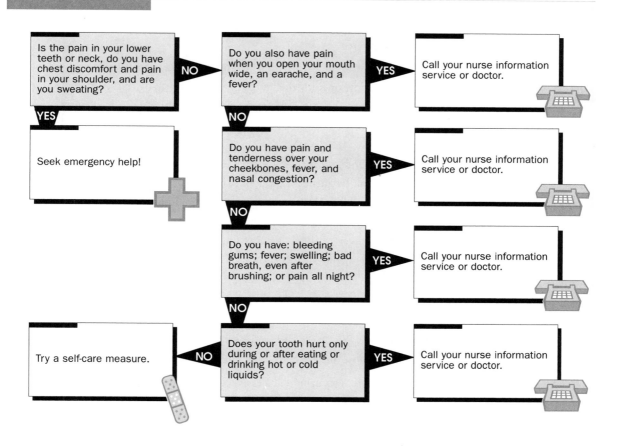

Is the pain in your lower teeth or neck, do you have chest discomfort and pain in your shoulder, and are you sweating?

NO → Do you also have pain when you open your mouth wide, an earache, and a fever?

YES → Call your nurse information service or doctor.

YES ↓

Seek emergency help!

NO ↓

Do you have pain and tenderness over your cheekbones, fever, and nasal congestion?

YES → Call your nurse information service or doctor.

NO ↓

Do you have: bleeding gums; fever; swelling; bad breath, even after brushing; or pain all night?

YES → Call your nurse information service or doctor.

NO ↓

Try a self-care measure.

NO ← Does your tooth hurt only during or after eating or drinking hot or cold liquids?

YES → Call your nurse information service or doctor.

Self-Care Measures

- Use ice packs and aspirin (don't use aspirin if you are under age 19), ibuprofen (*see* page 27), or another pain reliever.
- Don't ignore the pain.
- Don't ever suck on aspirin or place it on an aching tooth; aspirin should be swallowed whole and followed with plenty of water.
- You may use toothpaste for sensitive teeth, but be sure to carefully follow the package instructions for use (i.e., use only for a limited time and see your dentist if the pain lasts or worsens).

Prevention

- Brush and floss regularly (morning and night), according to your dentist's instructions (*see* figures).
- Avoid snacks, especially sweets, or keep them to a bare minimum. If you do snack, choose nuts or cheese, which neutralize the acid formation triggered by sugar. But remember, these foods are high in fat.

URINATION PROBLEM

The Problem

You feel pain, burning, or discomfort when urinating. Your urine is discolored, cloudy, or foul-smelling. You pass abnormally large or small amounts of urine. You can't urinate at all or you urinate too frequently.

Causes of Urination Problems

Infection (kidney, bladder, urinary tract, or urethra). You have burning during urination, frequent and urgent urination with only small amounts of urine passed, blood in the urine, lower abdominal pain, pain during intercourse or ejaculation, or a slight fever. You may have sudden fever and shaking chills; severe fatigue; burning and frequent urination with cloudy, bloody, or foul-smelling urine; or nausea and vomiting. You may have one of several kinds of infections. Women are especially likely to have urinary tract infections (UTIs); they should follow self-care measures along with prescribed treatment.

Blocked urethra. You have sudden urges to urinate but cannot pass any urine. This is most often seen in men and is potentially serious.

Hypopituitarism. You urinate excessively, feel tired and extremely thirsty, and have dry skin, chronic headaches, a decreased sex drive, and an intolerance to cold. Hypopituitarism is caused by underactivity of the pituitary gland, which secretes hormones that regulate the body's *metabolism.*

Sexually transmitted disease. You have pain or burning pain during urination, along with various other symptoms, including pain during intercourse, pus-like discharge from your penis or vagina, and itching around your genital area. These symptoms could suggest herpes (*see* page 42), *chlamydia, gonorrhea,* or some other sexually transmitted disease. If you have a sexually transmitted disease, avoid sexual contact until you've completed treatment. Any sexual partners in recent months should be informed.

Other Causes

Diabetes mellitus (*see* page 240)
Hormonal disorder
Prostate problem (*see* page 254)
Vaginitis
Excess fluid intake, especially caffeinated drinks or alcohol
Bladder *tumor*
Kidney stone (*see* page 204)
Kidney *gravel*

Treating Your Child

- See *Self-Care Measures* and *Prevention* listed here.

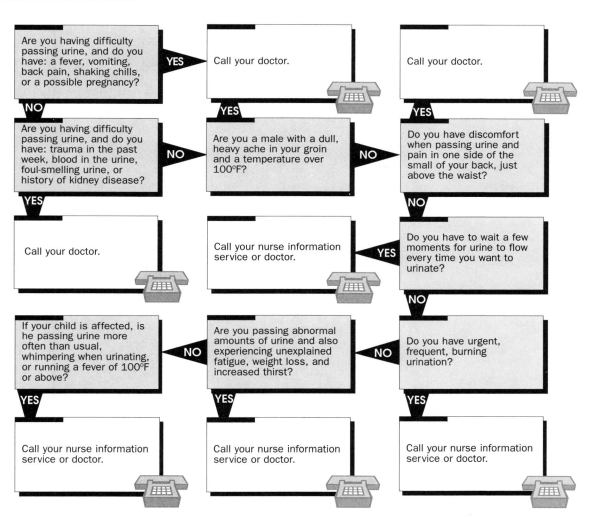

Are you having difficulty passing urine, and do you have: a fever, vomiting, back pain, shaking chills, or a possible pregnancy?

YES → Call your doctor.

NO

Are you having difficulty passing urine, and do you have: trauma in the past week, blood in the urine, foul-smelling urine, or history of kidney disease?

NO → Are you a male with a dull, heavy ache in your groin and a temperature over 100°F?

YES → Call your doctor.

YES

Call your doctor.

Call your nurse information service or doctor.

Do you have discomfort when passing urine and pain in one side of the small of your back, just above the waist?

YES → Call your doctor.

NO → Do you have to wait a few moments for urine to flow every time you want to urinate?

YES → Call your nurse information service or doctor.

NO

If your child is affected, is he passing urine more often than usual, whimpering when urinating, or running a fever of 100°F or above?

NO → Are you passing abnormal amounts of urine and also experiencing unexplained fatigue, weight loss, and increased thirst?

NO → Do you have urgent, frequent, burning urination?

YES

Call your nurse information service or doctor.

YES

Call your nurse information service or doctor.

YES

Call your nurse information service or doctor.

Self-Care Measures

- If you are experiencing symptoms of bladder infection (e.g., urgent, frequent burning urination, blood in the urine, low-grade fever, or pain in the lower abdomen or lower back), drink lots of fluids, especially cranberry juice and other fruit juices.

- If you are a woman who has frequent urinary tract infections, always wipe from front to back after a bowel movement or urinating. Urinate after sexual intercourse. Avoid bubble baths, perfumed soaps, or douches. Drink plenty of fluids, especially cranberry juice, and avoid caffeine.

Prevention

- If you have frequent urination, especially at night, cut down on the amount of tea, coffee, caffeinated sodas, or alcohol that you drink in the evening.

- Drinking cranberry juice may help prevent urinary tract infections.

203

URINE, BLOOD IN

The Problem

Your urine is reddish, pink, or brown, or contains red streaks or clots. Color pigments in food (e.g., beets), drug use, and *porphyria* can all cause urine to turn red. This is of no concern.

Causes of Blood in Urine

Bladder infection. You have urgent, painful, frequent, not very productive urination with blood in the urine, a fever, and lower back and pelvic pain. Bladder infections, or cystitis, are among the most common causes of incontinence and are treated with antibiotics.

Bladder stone. You have blood in your urine. You urinate often but pass little urine, and only when you're in a certain position; you have pain in your lower back and abdomen, with a low-grade fever.

Kidney stone. You have spasms of pain in your lower back, spreading to your lower abdomen and groin, and you have an urge to urinate but only pass a small amount of urine, with blood in it.

Urethritis. You have a yellowish discharge from the *urethra*, lower abdominal pain, and a frequent need to urinate, but pass only small amounts of urine that has blood in it. You also have a burning sensation when urinating and, if you are a woman, sexual intercourse is painful. Urethritis is caused by a bacterial infection which may be sexually transmitted or may result from poor personal hygiene.

Glomerulonephritis. Your bloody urine may be accompanied by swelling of your ankles or around your eyes, shortness of breath, and fatigue. You may have a sudden or chronic inflammation of the structures in your kidneys that filter blood.

Benign hematuria. You have blood in your urine and no other symptoms. This condition isn't associated with any illness or damage to

Treating Your Child

- See *Self-Care Measures* and *Prevention* listed here.

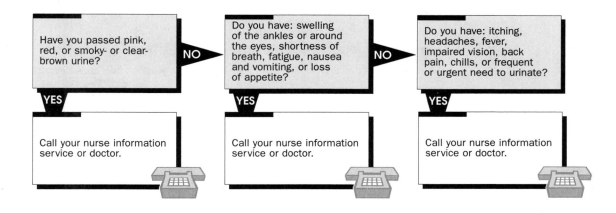

Have you passed pink, red, or smoky- or clear-brown urine?

NO →

Do you have: swelling of the ankles or around the eyes, shortness of breath, fatigue, nausea and vomiting, or loss of appetite?

NO →

Do you have: itching, headaches, fever, impaired vision, back pain, chills, or frequent or urgent need to urinate?

YES ↓ Call your nurse information service or doctor.

YES ↓ Call your nurse information service or doctor.

YES ↓ Call your nurse information service or doctor.

any organs, although urine may seem bloodier when you are suffering from viral infections (e.g., a cold). It sometimes appears in childhood and disappears with time. Occasionally, several members of a family develop this symptom, which may last for a lifetime but cause no problems.

Hemolytic anemia. You are tired and feel weak, there is blood in your urine, you are short of breath, and your skin may be jaundiced (i.e., yellow in color). Hemolytic anemia is caused by a genetic abnormality in the red blood cells or certain drugs or infectious diseases which destroy red blood cells. Red blood cells are destroyed and the bone marrow cannot produce replacement cells quickly enough. For people who have a genetic deficiency of a certain enzyme, certain medications may trigger hemolytic anemia.

Self-Care Measures

- If you have blood in your urine, you require treatment by a health-care professional.

Prevention

- Keep yourself well hydrated, drink at least 6 to 8 glasses of fluids a day; this is especially important when exercising, if you have a fever, or in hot weather.
- Avoid caffeine and alcohol, which may irritate the bladder.
- To avoid infections, always use latex condoms during sexual intercourse.
- Take showers instead of baths, and use mild soaps.

VAGINAL BLEEDING

The Problem

You have bleeding between menstrual periods, during pregnancy, or after menopause.

Causes of Vaginal Bleeding

Menopause. You're over 38, and you find that your periods are coming more frequently than usual or that you're having unexpected bleeding after a few months of no periods at all. This kind of irregular bleeding is quite normal in women at any time between their late 30s and early 50s (or earlier or later, for some women). It's a sign that menopause—the end of your monthly menstrual periods—is approaching. You may want to call your nurse information service or doctor and ask whether hormone replacement therapy is a good idea for you once you actually reach menopause. Otherwise, an occasional irregular period during this phase of your life is no cause for concern.

Birth control device. You have unexpected vaginal bleeding, and you've recently had an intrauterine device (IUD) inserted for birth control, or you're taking birth control pills. Both of these birth control methods may cause spotting between periods. This bleeding is unlikely to be a cause for concern.

Miscarriage. You are pregnant, and you have bleeding. Bleeding during pregnancy may be a sign of miscarriage, although some women experience bleeding throughout pregnancy.

Ectopic pregnancy. You have bleeding along with abdominal pain, and you're pregnant or in the very early stages of pregnancy. Bleeding early in pregnancy that's accompanied by abdominal pain may be a sign of an ectopic pregnancy, or a pregnancy developing outside the uterus (*see* figure). It requires emergency surgery to terminate the pregnancy.

Treating Your Child

- During the first 3 years of menstruation, an occasional irregular period is normal.

- In children, vaginal bleeding can sometimes be a sign of sexual molestation whether or not menstruation has begun.

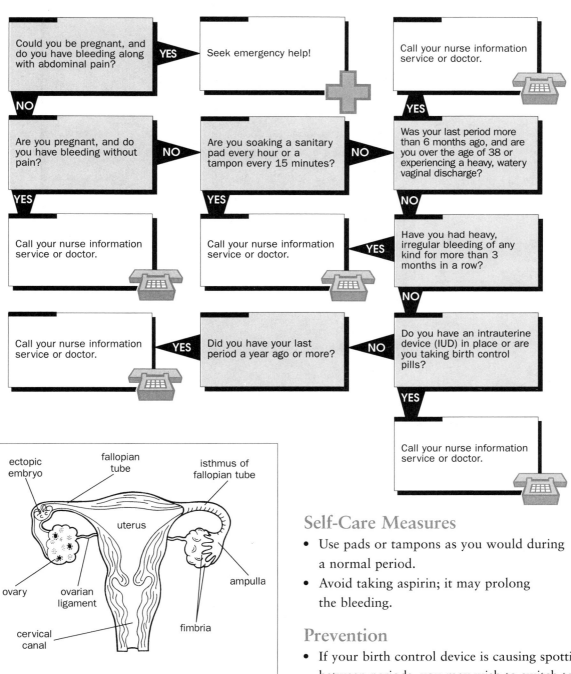

Could you be pregnant, and do you have bleeding along with abdominal pain?

YES → Seek emergency help!

NO ↓

Are you pregnant, and do you have bleeding without pain?

NO → Are you soaking a sanitary pad every hour or a tampon every 15 minutes?

NO → Was your last period more than 6 months ago, and are you over the age of 38 or experiencing a heavy, watery vaginal discharge?

YES → Call your nurse information service or doctor.

YES ↓ Call your nurse information service or doctor.

YES ↓ Call your nurse information service or doctor.

NO ↓

Have you had heavy, irregular bleeding of any kind for more than 3 months in a row?

YES → Call your nurse information service or doctor.

NO ↓

Do you have an intrauterine device (IUD) in place or are you taking birth control pills?

NO → Did you have your last period a year ago or more?

YES → Call your nurse information service or doctor.

YES ↓ Call your nurse information service or doctor.

Ectopic Pregnancy

ectopic embryo
fallopian tube
isthmus of fallopian tube
uterus
ampulla
ovary
ovarian ligament
cervical canal
fimbria

Self-Care Measures

- Use pads or tampons as you would during a normal period.
- Avoid taking aspirin; it may prolong the bleeding.

Prevention

- If your birth control device is causing spotting between periods, you may wish to switch to another method.

207

VAGINAL DISCHARGE/ITCH

The Problem

You have vaginal itching or excessive, discolored, foul-smelling discharge.

Causes of Vaginal Discharge and Itch

Other Causes

Sexually transmitted disease
 (*see* page 202)
Diabetes mellitus (*see* page 240)
Allergy
Menopause (*see* page 206)

Yeast infection. You have a thick, white, cheesy discharge, and irritation and itching around the vagina. A yeast infection is a fungal infection that often develops after taking antibiotics or birth control pills, or during pregnancy.

Forgotten tampon or diaphragm. You have an offensive discharge but no other symptoms. Check for a forgotten tampon or diaphragm.

Pelvic inflammatory disease/salpingitis. You may have a discolored, foul-smelling vaginal discharge and/or pelvic pain. You may also have a low-grade fever and chills, fatigue, low-back pain, irregular menstrual bleeding, and loss of appetite. Pelvic inflammatory disease and salpingitis, an infection of your fallopian tubes, require immediate medical attention.

Self-Care Measures

- Do not douche unless advised by your doctor.
- If you have vaginal itching, avoid scratching, and wash twice a day with plain water. Wear cotton underpants, and avoid pantyhose and tight jeans or slacks. Sleep without underpants.

Treating Your Child

- Vaginal discharge is unusual in girls before puberty. In such a case, sexual abuse should be considered and discussed with your doctor.
- To make your child more comfortable, try these measures:
  - Gently wash the area twice a day with plain water.
  - Have her wear cotton underpants only. Launder them with perfume-free, additive-free detergents.
  - Teach her to wipe from front to back after using the toilet.

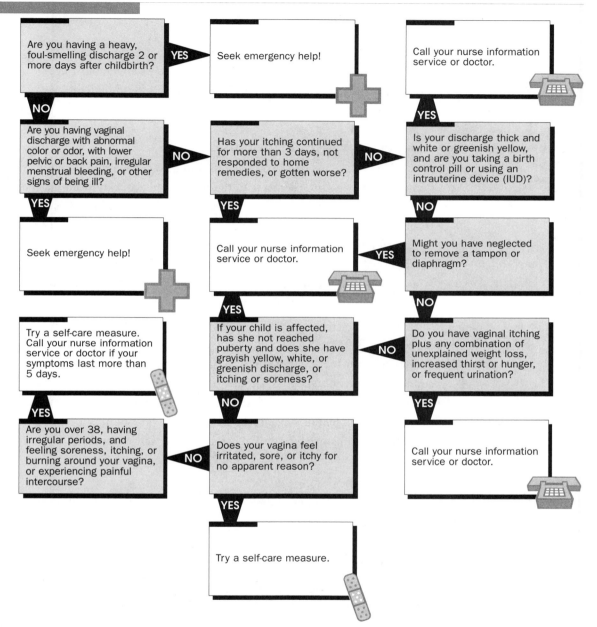

Are you having a heavy, foul-smelling discharge 2 or more days after childbirth?

YES → Seek emergency help!

NO ↓

Are you having vaginal discharge with abnormal color or odor, with lower pelvic or back pain, irregular menstrual bleeding, or other signs of being ill?

NO → Has your itching continued for more than 3 days, not responded to home remedies, or gotten worse?

YES ↓

Seek emergency help!

Call your nurse information service or doctor.

Try a self-care measure. Call your nurse information service or doctor if your symptoms last more than 5 days.

If your child is affected, has she not reached puberty and does she have grayish yellow, white, or greenish discharge, or itching or soreness?

YES ↓

Are you over 38, having irregular periods, and feeling soreness, itching, or burning around your vagina, or experiencing painful intercourse?

NO → Does your vagina feel irritated, sore, or itchy for no apparent reason?

YES ↓

Try a self-care measure.

Call your nurse information service or doctor.

Is your discharge thick and white or greenish yellow, and are you taking a birth control pill or using an intrauterine device (IUD)?

YES ↑ Call your nurse information service or doctor.

NO ↓

Might you have neglected to remove a tampon or diaphragm?

YES → Call your nurse information service or doctor.

NO ↓

Do you have vaginal itching plus any combination of unexplained weight loss, increased thirst or hunger, or frequent urination?

YES ↓

Call your nurse information service or doctor.

Prevention

- Safe sex and latex condoms for male sex partners will help prevent some sexually transmitted diseases.

- If you're prone to yeast infections, use an over-the-counter anti-yeast preparation if you're taking an antibiotic. Eating yogurt with live active cultures may also help.

209

VISION PROBLEM

The Problem

Your ability to see has worsened. This change may include blurring, diminished field of vision, or seeing double images, flashing lights, or floating spots.

Other Causes

Glaucoma (*see* page 230)
Cataract (*see* page 230)
Stroke (*see* page 258)
Concussion
Eyestrain (*see* page 88)
Refraction error
Eye infection
Eye inflammation
Migraine (*see* page 112)
Medication side effect
Diabetes (*see* page 240)
Exophthalmos
Retinal detachment
Macular degeneration
Optic neuritis

Causes of Vision Problems

Aging. You're over 50, and you've noticed that you have to hold your book farther away in order to read the print. You've also noticed that you're occasionally seeing little spots that look like swarming gnats in front of your eyes. Visual changes do occur with age, and most of them are nothing to be concerned about. It's not unusual, for example, for older people to see "floaters"—little black spots that seem to drift into your field of vision. They're nothing more than harmless bits of your eyeball's inner fluid floating into view. However, the sudden appearance of numerous floaters could mean a more serious eye problem and needs to be investigated.

Brain hemorrhage. You have blurred or double vision accompanied by sudden loss of consciousness; sudden, severe headache; paralysis on one side of your face or body; weakness or dizziness; confusion; and/or loss of speech. Brain hemorrhage, or bleeding within the brain, is a very rare cause of visual disturbance, but it's an extremely serious one.

Treating Your Child

- Children may not be verbal enough to tell you when they're having visual problems. If your child's vision suddenly seems to change—if he blinks or squints often or complains of not being able to see the blackboard, for example, or if he doesn't seem to recognize familiar people from several feet away—call your nurse information service or doctor.

- A child with a "lazy eye" may have an eye that wanders, especially when tired. Call your nurse information service or doctor for more information.

- A child who always watches TV with his head turned to one side may have a problem with his other eye.

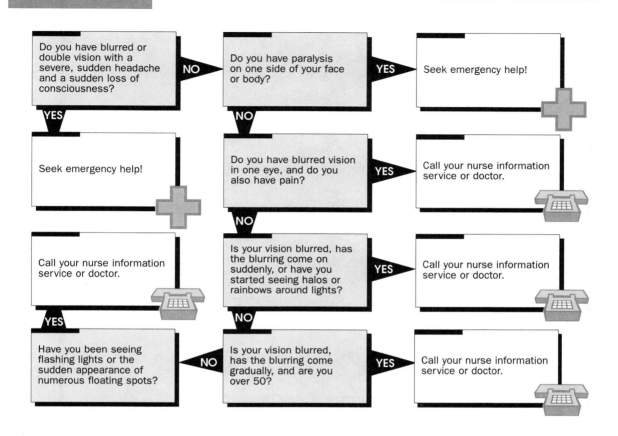

Do you have blurred or double vision with a severe, sudden headache and a sudden loss of consciousness?

NO → Do you have paralysis on one side of your face or body?

YES → Seek emergency help!

YES ↓

Seek emergency help!

NO ↓

Do you have blurred vision in one eye, and do you also have pain?

YES → Call your nurse information service or doctor.

Call your nurse information service or doctor.

NO ↓

Is your vision blurred, has the blurring come on suddenly, or have you started seeing halos or rainbows around lights?

YES → Call your nurse information service or doctor.

YES ↓

Have you been seeing flashing lights or the sudden appearance of numerous floating spots?

NO ← Is your vision blurred, has the blurring come gradually, and are you over 50?

YES → Call your nurse information service or doctor.

Self-Care Measures

- If your visual disturbances are caused by eye strain (e.g., the result of long hours spent in front of a computer screen or reading small print), rest is all that you need. If you can't lie down and close your eyes, at least shift your gaze. Look out the window for a while, or take a walk. Try to shift your focus from close eye work several times an hour to avoid eye fatigue.

- If you're seeing floaters, try rapidly moving your eyes up and down. This action stirs up the eyeballs' fluid, causing the floaters to settle outside your line of vision.

Prevention

- Since many eye problems increase in frequency with age, it's important to have your eyes checked regularly—about once a year—after age 50.

WART

The Problem

You have a small, raised, rough bump on your skin that is the same color as the surrounding skin or slightly darker. The bump is painless and doesn't itch.

Important Information About Warts

Warts are an extremely common skin condition. Many are harmless (genital and anal warts are an exception), and most disappear within 2 years. Warts are caused by the human papilloma virus (HPV), of which there are more than 60 types. The virus is mildly contagious and enters the skin through tiny breaks in its surface. You can catch warts from other people. Common warts most often appear on the hands and fingers; plantar warts appear on the soles of the feet; periungual warts are found around the fingernails and toenails; digitate warts are small, fingerlike projections that are located on the scalp; and flat warts cluster in groups of as many as several hundred. Genital and anal warts (i.e., small, fleshy growths in your genital or anal area) result from sexual transmission of HPV. Do not use self-care measures to treat genital and anal warts.

Self-Care Measures

- Wart removal preparations containing salicylic or lactic acid are available over the counter in drugstores and supermarkets; they can be very effective. Follow the package directions exactly. Don't use wart removers on your face. Do not use wart removers on any area that is infected or reddened, or if you have diabetes or poor blood circulation.

Prevention

- Don't bite or pick at warts; doing so can cause them to spread to other areas of your skin.

Treating Your Child

- Warts are more common in teenagers and children than in adults. Reassure your child that warts are nothing serious, and unless they are on the bottom of the feet and causing pain, consider waiting for them to go away on their own.

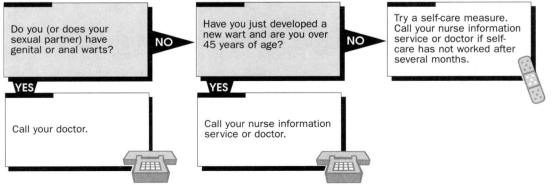

Do you (or does your sexual partner) have genital or anal warts?

NO → Have you just developed a new wart and are you over 45 years of age?

NO → Try a self-care measure. Call your nurse information service or doctor if self-care has not worked after several months.

YES → Call your doctor.

YES → Call your nurse information service or doctor.

WEIGHT GAIN

The Problem

You've steadily or suddenly gained weight without having changed your eating or exercise patterns.

Other Causes

Depression (*see* page 238)
Stress (*see* page 23)

Causes of Weight Gain

Medication side effect. You've gained weight after starting to take steroids, cortisone drugs, oral contraceptives, or nonsteroidal anti-inflammatory drugs (NSAIDs, which include over-the-counter preparations).

Edema. You have gained weight and feel "thick." Your ankles, legs, or abdomen may be swollen. You may also be urinating less (or urinating much more during the night). You may be suffering from fluid accumulation in your tissues due to congestive heart failure (*see* page 234) or kidney disease. These are life-threatening conditions.

Treating Your Child

- If your child is gaining weight more rapidly than standard growth charts suggest is normal, *see* page 249.

Self-Care Measures

- If you've recently quit smoking: Exercise more than you have in the past, eat a balanced diet, drink plenty of water, and avoid compulsive eating as a substitute for smoking.
- Balance your diet (*see* page 17). Emphasize fresh vegetables and fruits, then grains, then proteins; keep fats in check. Avoid alcohol, sugar, sweetened fruit drinks or colas, nuts, potato chips, and pastries. Exercise.

Prevention

- Don't smoke (*see* page 24). Eat a healthy, balanced diet.

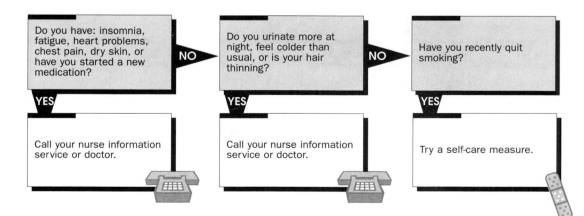

Do you have: insomnia, fatigue, heart problems, chest pain, dry skin, or have you started a new medication?

NO → Do you urinate more at night, feel colder than usual, or is your hair thinning?

NO → Have you recently quit smoking?

YES — Call your nurse information service or doctor.

YES — Call your nurse information service or doctor.

YES — Try a self-care measure.

WEIGHT LOSS

The Problem

You've lost weight suddenly or without trying.

Other Causes

Diabetes mellitus (*see* page 240)
Anorexia nervosa (*see* page 35)
Tumor
Depression (*see* page 238)
Stress (*see* page 23)

Causes of Weight Loss

Nutrient malabsorption. You may have foul-smelling, yellowish diarrhea, abdominal cramps, bloating, weakness, and lethargy that have lasted over 2 weeks. Your small intestine has a problem absorbing the nutrients in your diet.

Chronic infection. You have weight loss plus drenching night sweats, recurring fever, persistent or bloody cough, and a general feeling of being ill. These symptoms could be due to *tuberculosis, brucellosis*, AIDS (*see* page 242), or other serious chronic conditions.

Treating Your Child

- See *Self-Care Measures* and *Prevention* listed here.

Self-Care Measures

- Any unexplained weight loss requires medical evaluation and advice.

Prevention

- To prevent nutrient malabsorption, the underlying cause must be treated. Causes include infection, cardiovascular problems, medications, and laxatives.

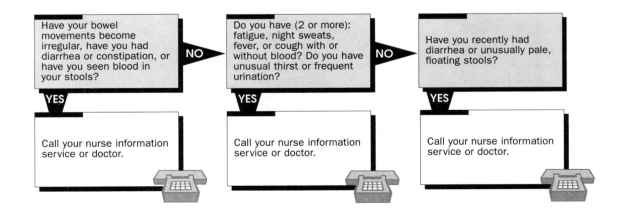

Have your bowel movements become irregular, have you had diarrhea or constipation, or have you seen blood in your stools? **NO**

Do you have (2 or more): fatigue, night sweats, fever, or cough with or without blood? Do you have unusual thirst or frequent urination? **NO**

Have you recently had diarrhea or unusually pale, floating stools?

YES → Call your nurse information service or doctor.

YES → Call your nurse information service or doctor.

YES → Call your nurse information service or doctor.

WOUND, PUNCTURE

The Problem

You have an injury caused by a sharp, pointed object, such as a nail, pin, tack, needle, staple, or wire.

Important Information About Puncture Wounds

The primary concern with puncture wounds is infection. The object that caused the wound can carry disease-causing organisms deep into the skin. Signs of infection will not begin to appear until about 24 hours after the injury has occurred. Report any puncture wound to your nurse information service or doctor, even if you believe you've cleaned it thoroughly and the puncture has bled freely. Because it can take so long for the signs of infection to show up, your doctor may start you on antibiotics right away to avoid any complications. You may also need a tetanus booster shot.

Treating Your Child

- See *Self-Care Measures* on page 65 and *Prevention* listed here.

Self-Care Measures

- For information on self-care, *see* page 65.

Prevention

- Puncture wounds to the bottoms of feet are very common. To avoid them, wear shoes when outside, and see that your children do the same.

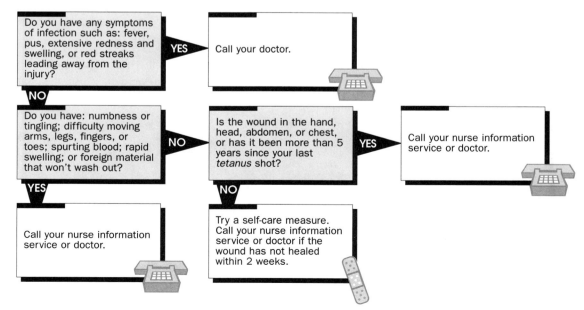

Do you have any symptoms of infection such as: fever, pus, extensive redness and swelling, or red streaks leading away from the injury?

YES → Call your doctor.

NO ↓

Do you have: numbness or tingling; difficulty moving arms, legs, fingers, or toes; spurting blood; rapid swelling; or foreign material that won't wash out?

NO → Is the wound in the hand, head, abdomen, or chest, or has it been more than 5 years since your last *tetanus* shot?

YES → Call your nurse information service or doctor.

YES ↓ Call your nurse information service or doctor.

NO ↓ Try a self-care measure. Call your nurse information service or doctor if the wound has not healed within 2 weeks.

WRIST PAIN

The Problem

You have pain and possibly numbness and tingling in one or both wrists.

Other Causes

Tendinitis (*see* page 174)
Arthritis (*see* page 224)
Infection
Osteoporosis (*see* page 250)
Cyst

Causes of Wrist Pain

Carpal tunnel syndrome. You have numbness, tingling, and pain in your wrist, thumb, and first three fingers, and possibly in half of your fourth (i.e., ring) finger as well. The pain may shoot up your arm from your wrist. Your symptoms are worse at night and may be severe enough to wake you from sleep; however, if you hang your hand over the side of the bed and shake it, the pain lessens. If it lasts long enough, you may have hand weakness.

Carpal tunnel syndrome occurs when the *tendons* between your arm and hand become inflamed and swollen and begin to close in on the major nerve of the wrist. Carpal tunnel syndrome is especially common among people who do repetitive work or activity with their hands, such as typing, assembly-line work, knitting, golfing, or sewing. Hormonal changes due to pregnancy or menopause (*see* page 206), diabetes mellitus (*see* page 240), or hypothyroidism (*see* page 127) may also increase the risk of this syndrome. Carpal tunnel syndrome often goes away on its own, and self-care measures may also help a great deal. However, in some cases, surgery may be necessary to prevent permanent nerve damage.

Wrist injury. You have pain and throbbing in your wrist, probably after falling on your outstretched hand. You may also notice a clicking or grinding sound coming from the joint. Sprains and strains (*see* page 182) are the most common wrist injuries, but *fractures* can occur

Treating Your Child

- Follow the self-care measures listed here if your child injures his wrist. However, don't give aspirin to anyone under 19 years of age! It may cause a rare but serious problem called Reye's syndrome. Instead, use ibuprofen or acetaminophen (*see* page 27) for fever or pain.

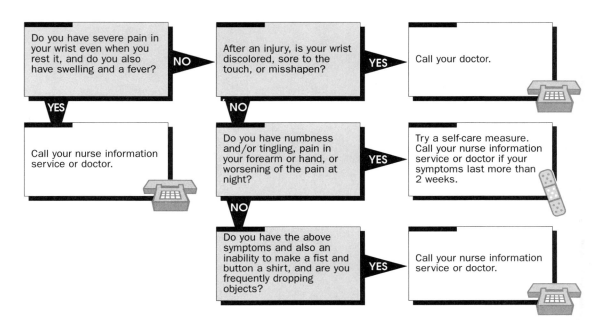

Do you have severe pain in your wrist even when you rest it, and do you also have swelling and a fever? — **NO** →

After an injury, is your wrist discolored, sore to the touch, or misshapen? — **YES** → Call your doctor.

YES ↓
Call your nurse information service or doctor.

NO ↓
Do you have numbness and/or tingling, pain in your forearm or hand, or worsening of the pain at night? — **YES** → Try a self-care measure. Call your nurse information service or doctor if your symptoms last more than 2 weeks.

NO ↓
Do you have the above symptoms and also an inability to make a fist and button a shirt, and are you frequently dropping objects? — **YES** → Call your nurse information service or doctor.

in any of the small bones of the wrist.

Infection. You have pain in your wrist, along with swelling that developed rapidly and a fever of 101°F or higher. You will need antibiotics if your wrist is infected.

Self-Care Measures

- If carpal tunnel syndrome is the problem, rest is crucial to protecting your wrist from further damage. For example, if your wrist pain is caused by typing or keyboarding all day, try to stop for 1 or 2 weeks; if that's not possible, at least take frequent rest breaks.
- Splint your wrists so that they remain stable. Buy a splint from a drugstore or medical-supply house, and wear it constantly for 3 or 4 days, then just at night for a few more weeks.
- If your wrist pain is caused by an injury, elevate the wrist, and apply a cold pack to the area to decrease pain and swelling for the first

24 to 48 hours. Apply warm, moist heat (for 15 to 20 minutes, 3 times a day) after 48 to 72 hours and once the swelling has gone down. Wrap an elastic bandage around your wrist (securely, but not too tightly) to reduce swelling and to help protect the injured area.

- Try an over-the-counter pain reliever, preferably aspirin or ibuprofen (*see* page 27), since they can also help to reduce inflammation.

Prevention

- You can help prevent carpal tunnel syndrome by taking frequent breaks from any strenuous work or activity that requires repetitive hand motions and by varying your movements so that your wrists are not constantly bent. Using a wrist-support pad (available in many office-supply stores) while typing or keyboarding may also help.

UNDERSTANDING LONG-TERM AILMENTS

ALCOHOLISM

What is alcoholism?

Alcoholism is a chronic (i.e., long-lasting) disease marked by the inability to control consumption of alcohol. The disease may begin when people drink to relieve stress, but it progresses when they start drinking simply to feel normal. In time, they experience uncontrollable cravings for alcohol and suffer from recurring alcohol-related troubles: damaged relationships with family and friends, inability to function at work, financial difficulties, encounters with the law, or serious medical problems.

What causes alcoholism?

Alcoholism is not a fault, moral failing, or spiritual weakness. Instead, it is a complex physical illness resulting from a combination of factors. The disease tends to run in families. Perhaps half of all alcoholics inherit a genetic susceptibility to the illness. People who suffer from psychiatric illnesses, such as depression (*see* page 238) or a personality disorder, often abuse alcohol. Social and cultural pressures are also involved. A person who lives with an alcoholic or whose family relationships are seriously disturbed is more likely to develop alcoholism. Other cases arise from unknown causes.

What are the symptoms of alcoholism?

The symptoms of alcoholism usually worsen over time. Three drinking patterns commonly seen among alcoholics are regular, daily intoxication; use of large amounts of alcohol at specific times; and long periods of sobriety interspersed with drinking binges lasting weeks or months.

In the early stages, an alcoholic may appear to be a fun-loving person who simply drinks too much on social occasions or who drinks to relieve fatigue, depression, or anxiety. In time, the person may experience blackouts—waking in the morning with no memory of events from the previous night. As the problem becomes more obvious, the person becomes more secretive about drinking: hiding bottles, sneaking liquor into other beverages, lying about activities. Typically, people with alcoholism vehemently deny there's a problem, or they promise they'll stop drinking. Eventually the disease makes people feel depressed, resentful, guilty, or afraid.

Many alcoholics have distinctive physical traits: a flushed, veiny appearance (especially of the nose); bruises; and trembling hands. Loss of muscle control, dizziness, and impaired judgment make them susceptible to falls and accidents. Destruction of brain cells leads to loss of memory and concentration and personality changes. Other medical illnesses may develop, such as cirrhosis of the liver (i.e., progressive liver disease which eventually results in liver failure), *gastritis*, neuropathy, and malnutrition. In extreme cases, people experience delirium tremens, or the "D.T.'s," marked by trembling, confusion, and hallucinations. Alcoholism is often fatal.

Can alcoholism be prevented?

Alcohol is a legal drug, easily obtained and heavily promoted in the media. People who know they are susceptible to alcoholism or who have a family history of alcoholism should moderate their consumption. If they feel unable to control their drinking, they should speak to a medical professional, counselor, or clergy member. Local and national organizations (e.g., Alcoholics Anonymous [AA], Al-Anon, and Al-Ateen) provide counseling and support for alcoholics and their loved ones. Pregnant women should not drink at all to avoid risk of damage to the fetus.

How is alcoholism treated?

Alcoholism, like other diseases such as diabetes, cannot be cured, but it can be treated. The goal of treatment is total abstinence. In some cases, the alcoholic seeks help only after "hitting bottom"—experiencing a complication such as financial disaster, abandonment by loved ones, or serious injury. More often, though, alcoholics need to be confronted by concerned friends or relatives who insist that they get help.

Some people recover following a short stay in a detoxification center in a hospital or clinic, where trained experts provide a safe and reassuring environment while helping them deal with the devastating symptoms of withdrawal from alcohol. Rehabilitation centers or hospitals offer long-term care. Such programs offer treatment for other problems, such as anxiety or malnutrition; provide group and individual therapy sessions; and make referrals to support groups, such as AA. Treatment may require hospitalization, but many people do well as outpatients. Some people in treatment benefit from a drug called Antabuse, which causes them to become violently ill if they take even a sip of alcohol.

Because recurrence of alcoholism is always just a sip away, the process of recovery is a lifetime responsibility, a never-ending day-to-day

commitment. For this reason, people in recovery need strong support once they leave the hospital or treatment program. Millions of people have benefited from taking part in AA meetings or similar programs. Through professional therapy, they can learn new patterns of thinking and behavior to help them avoid the pitfalls of the past. Members of the family may also need training to learn how to help their loved ones recover. Additional treatment can address other associated problems, such as underlying psychiatric or physical illnesses.

When to seek help.

Seek emergency help if:

- You drink so much that you experience blackouts or have alcohol-related accidents.

Call your nurse information service or doctor if:

- You experience strong cravings for alcohol or feel you have a problem with the amount that you drink.

ALZHEIMER'S DISEASE

What is Alzheimer's disease?

Alzheimer's disease (also called Alzheimer's dementia) is a condition in which brain cells deteriorate and die. The brain loses the ability to process new information or store and retrieve memories. For this reason, it is physically impossible for people in later stages of Alzheimer's to learn or retain new things, or remember even the most important facts, events, and people in their lives. Alzheimer's grows steadily worse as time passes.

What causes Alzheimer's disease?

Researchers have not yet identified the cause of Alzheimer's. Some people inherit a genetic weakness. There is no conclusive evidence that metals, such as aluminum, play a role.

Is Alzheimer's disease different from other forms of dementia?

Dementia is a general term meaning loss of brain function. About 80% of people with dementia have Alzheimer's, which damages brain cells in a specific and telltale way. In making a diagnosis, doctors look for other conditions that may be causing dementia-like symptoms, such as a vitamin deficiency, depression (*see* page 238), low blood sugar, or abnormal fluid pressure on the brain.

Senile dementia is brain cell loss in the elderly resulting from a disease process similar to Alzheimer's, but occurring at an advanced age. The symptoms are similar: loss of memory, mental confusion, inability to function, and under the microscope, the brain tissue looks the same.

Dementia can occur due to repeated stroke (*see* page 258), when blocked *arteries* in the brain destroy cells responsible for *cognitive functioning*, but dementia is not an inevitable consequence of stroke. This condition is called multi-infarct dementia and results from blockages in many blood vessels over time. This causes loss of mental ability but typically not paralysis or other usual stroke symptoms.

Chronic abuse of alcohol (*see* page 220) and severe illnesses, such as AIDS (*see* page 242), or certain infectious diseases, can cause dementia in people of any age.

What are the symptoms of Alzheimer's disease?

The loss of mental function begins slowly and may continue for a decade or more. People forget dates, names, faces; they lose track of where they put things; they become irritable. Often they can't remember the most recent events or information—last week's birthday party, for example—but their older memories may seem especially vivid.

Over time, cognitive function ebbs, and they lose reasoning ability, use of language, coherent speech, judgment, and the capacity to understand or relate to their surroundings. Personality may change, leading to uncharacteristic behavior, and they may experience sudden mood swings, *hallucinations*, or *delusions*. In advanced stages, physical movement or speech may become difficult or impossible. People with the disease lose the ability to care for themselves; they may have poor hygiene and lose control over their bladder and bowel functions. Ultimately, Alzheimer's can cause death.

Can Alzheimer's disease be prevented?

There is no known way to prevent the onset of Alzheimer's disease.

How is Alzheimer's disease treated?

In less severe cases, a drug called Cognex may temporarily improve symptoms. Another drug, Hydergine, is sometimes given to promote blood circulation to the brain, but its effectiveness in treating Alzheimer's is largely unproven.

Other treatments are aimed at relieving symptoms related to dementia, such as insomnia, depression, delusions, or other psychiatric complaints. Such methods as dietary supplements with lecithin or the use of amphetamines or blood pressure medications have not proved helpful. Alzheimer's patients become easily confused and disoriented; consequently, routine and orienting cues are important. Maintain the same schedule of eating, bathing, napping, and sleeping every day; keep large clocks and calendars easily visible; keep a low light and quiet music on at night since this is usually the most difficult time for patients with Alzheimer's disease. Breaking the routine with a trip to an unfamiliar environment may prove disastrous.

What do families need to know about dealing with a person with Alzheimer's disease?

It helps to understand that Alzheimer's destroys brain cells, making it physically impossible for people with the disease to think, remember, or act the way they used to. Their behavior may be erratic, embarrassing, even dangerous, but it's important to remember such problems are caused by a serious disease and are not due to willfulness or ignorance.

Sometimes people with dementia wander off and become lost. Provide the person with an ID bracelet or card that indicates whom to call in case of emergency. In many cases, a person with Alzheimer's needs care around the clock. This can impose enormous burdens; families are sometimes referred to as the "other victims" of dementia. Family caregivers may need help in the form of psychological counseling, emotional support, or simply some time away from having to deal with the problem. Adult care centers can provide supervised care of the person for part or all of the day. There are many good resource materials available to educate you about this disease (e.g., *The 36-Hour Day: A Family Guide to Caring for Persons with Alzheimer's Disease, Related Dementing Illnesses, and Memory Loss in Later Life* by Nancy L. Mace and Peter V. Rabins, Warner Books, 1994, and *How to Care for Aging Parents* by Virginia Morris, Workman Publishing, 1996), and local support groups can also help.

When to seek help.

Call your nurse information service or doctor if:

- You notice increasingly frequent or severe memory lapses in an older relative.
- You notice persistent and unexplained personality or behavioral changes.

ARTHRITIS

What is arthritis?

Arthritis is a general term for a group of diseases involving pain, swelling, and stiffness in the joints, such as fingers, knees, or hips. The two main types are rheumatoid arthritis and osteoarthritis.

In rheumatoid arthritis, the membrane that surrounds the joint and produces the synovial membrane (i.e., a lubricating fluid) becomes inflamed, tender, and swollen, causing pain and stiffness.

Osteoarthritis (also called degenerative joint disease or "wear-and-tear" arthritis) is the most common form of arthritis, resulting when the protective layer of cartilage between bones wears down with use and with age. As bones rub together, they develop "spurs" (i.e., rough spots) that restrict movement and cause pain. In most cases, osteoarthritis is a less debilitating condition than rheumatoid arthritis.

What causes arthritis?

Rheumatoid arthritis is an autoimmune disease, which means the body's immune system mistakenly "attacks" its own tissue (in this case the synovial membrane) and causes inflammation. Why this happens is unknown, although flare-ups may be triggered by viruses or stress.

Osteoarthritis is a normal result of aging. Injury or repetitive overuse of the joints by people in certain occupations (e.g., athletes) can lead to osteoarthritis. Risk factors include heredity, obesity, previous joint disease, or other disorders that affect body shape and *metabolism*.

What are the symptoms of arthritis?

The main symptoms are pain and stiffness in the joints that are serious enough to restrict movement. As the disease worsens, the joints can become deformed; knobby areas may form on the fingers, especially in osteoarthritis.

A distinguishing feature of rheumatoid arthritis is inflammation, which causes the joints to become red, swollen, and warm to the touch. Pain and stiffness are typically most severe in the morning (the "gel" phenomenon) but improve during the day. The disease can affect any joint, but the fingers, toes, wrists, and knees are often involved, most often symmetrically on both sides of the body. Unlike osteoarthritis, rheumatoid arthritis seldom develops in the hips or spine (although involvement of the neck or cervical spine does occur and can cause serious consequences). Early in the disease, before joints become affected, many people experience such symptoms as fever, fatigue, loss of appetite, and morning stiffness. Over time, rheumatoid *nodules* (i.e., red, painless lumps) may appear just under the skin, especially on the elbow, although these can be seen elsewhere. Other symptoms include chest pain, difficulty breathing (due to pleurisy or lung involvement), dry mouth, and dry eyes.

Osteoarthritis tends to affect the end and middle joints of the fingers and the larger, weight-bearing joints in the hips, knees, and spine. It may develop on one or both sides of the body. Pain becomes worse with movement and gets better with rest; sometimes changes in the weather can trigger symptoms. Joints make an audible cracking noise when moved. Knobs often develop on the fingers. Only in rare cases is inflammation a symptom of osteoarthritis.

Can arthritis be prevented?

No one knows how to prevent rheumatoid arthritis. Strategies for preventing osteoarthritis include maintaining a healthy weight to minimize stress on joints and perhaps avoiding excessively repetitive joint movements.

How is arthritis treated?

There is no cure for arthritis. Goals of treatment are to reduce pain and inflammation and prevent loss of function. Nonsteroidal anti-inflammatory drugs (NSAIDs) (*see* page 28) are standard treatments. Aspirin (*see* page 27) relieves both pain and inflammation, but it must be taken at higher doses to achieve these effects. Because these drugs have potential adverse effects (e.g., stomach upset, bleeding, and kidney disease), always check with your nurse information service or doctor before taking any of these products, even the over-the-counter varieties.

Regular moderate exercise, especially swimming (in a heated pool, if possible), is important because people with arthritis naturally tend to restrict their movements, which can cause their muscles to waste away. Getting plenty of rest on a bed with a firm mattress and keeping your weight at a healthy level can help. No special diets have been shown to be of benefit in relieving arthritis. Avoid exercising—except for gentle, passive range-of-motion exercises—during flare-ups. Heat applied to the joints can be soothing (but should not be used if you're a diabetic or have impaired circulation), as can creams or lotions containing capsaicin or menthol. Some people benefit from temporary splints or braces that support the joint and give it a rest.

In more serious cases of rheumatoid arthritis, medications may be prescribed to relieve symptoms. Steroidal drugs injected directly into the joint provide quick, temporary relief for severe flare-ups. Surgery is also an option.

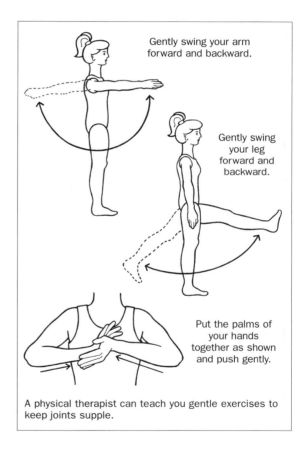

Gently swing your arm forward and backward.

Gently swing your leg forward and backward.

Put the palms of your hands together as shown and push gently.

A physical therapist can teach you gentle exercises to keep joints supple.

When to seek help.

Call your nurse information service or doctor if:

- Your joint pain is interfering with your normal activities, is severe, or won't go away.

ASTHMA

What is asthma?

Asthma is a chronic, episodic, reversible breathing disorder that occurs when the air passages in the lungs become inflamed in an immune response to an allergen or irritant. Inflammation causes tissues to swell, which narrows the airways and makes them oversensitive to irritation. Inflamed airways produce excess fluid (i.e., mucus), which clogs breathing passages. At the same time, the muscles surrounding the airways tighten. These factors combine to make breathing difficult.

What are the symptoms of asthma?

Common symptoms include wheezing; chest tightness; coughing, especially at night, in cold weather, or with exercise; shortness of breath; and excess mucus. In severe attacks, symptoms include rapid pulse, sweating, anxiety, gasping for breath, flaring nostrils, tightening of neck or chest muscles, bluish lips or fingertips, and exhaustion or confusion.

What causes asthma attacks?

Factors that can trigger asthma attacks include:

- Allergens such as dust and dust mites (i.e., tiny household parasites), pollen, mold, and dander from animals with fur or feathers
- Cigarette smoke, including secondhand smoke
- Chemical fumes
- Poor air quality
- Respiratory infections (e.g., colds, *influenza*, or *pneumonia*)
- Exercise
- Changes in weather, especially from mild to cold weather
- Certain medications
- Food additives, such as sulfites
- Cold drinks
- Emotional stress

How can asthma attacks be prevented?

To avoid allergens, clean your home once a week to reduce dust mites. Special vacuum cleaners with filters are available, or put 4 to 5 mothballs in standard vacuum bags. Remove fabrics that trap dust: Avoid thick rugs or wall-to-wall carpets (use area rugs or wood or tile floors), replace upholstered furniture with vinyl or wood, use shades or blinds instead of drapes, replace down pillows with synthetic fibers, and use pillow and mattress covers.

People with asthma should not smoke or be in a room with smokers (*see* page 24). Stay indoors as much as possible during very poor air quality days.

When possible, use air-conditioning. Change the filters monthly on air conditioners and furnaces.

If exercise or cold air triggers attacks, use medications before exercising or going outdoors. Wear a mask or scarf to warm the air before you breathe it. Swimming in a heated pool is generally well tolerated.

If your doctor recommends it, get immunized to prevent flu or pneumonia.

How can asthma be monitored?

The peak-flow meter, a simple handheld device that measures your ability to exhale, is an important tool for determining your normal breathing capacity (i.e., your "personal best"). Using the meter regularly—and recording the results in a diary—can both show whether your asthma is under control and warn if an attack is coming. If the reading is 60 to 80% of normal, use medicines as prescribed; if less than 60% of normal, call your nurse information service or doctor.

How is asthma treated?

Careful use of medications can reduce inflammation and reverse symptoms, thus preventing asthma attacks. There are several main types of medication, each providing a different and necessary action.

Anti-inflammatory drugs (especially steroids) prevent attacks by relieving the underlying airway inflammation and reducing sensitivity to asthma triggers. Usually these medications can be inhaled.

Bronchodilators treat symptoms of an attack. When inhaled, they open the narrowed airways. Some bronchodilators provide immediate short-term relief (2 to 4 hours). Other, newer drugs do not work as quickly, but can be used in advance to prevent symptoms for up to 12 hours and should not be repeated throughout the day. Always carry a bronchodilator with you.

Inhaled cromalyn (which prevents certain cells lining the bronchiole tree from releasing histamine, a chemical that causes airway narrowing) may be beneficial.

Additional treatments include oral drugs to prevent nighttime flare-ups (e.g., theophyllines). People whose asthma is allergy-related may receive immunotherapy, which attempts to build up the body's resistance to allergic triggers. Staying well hydrated is beneficial, especially during an attack.

Correct use of an inhaler

Shake the canister to mix the medicine. Exhale fully. Then release the dose while slowly inhaling. Breathe deeply so the medicine can reach the lungs' airways. Hold your breath as long as you can, for at least 10 seconds. Wait 30 seconds before taking the second dose. Rinse your mouth after use.

Using a spacer device—a plastic chamber which attaches to the inhaler and delivers the aerosol with less force—makes it easier to breathe medicine directly into the lungs without spraying it onto the back of the throat, where it may be swallowed. Spacers are of particular use to those who have trouble coordinating their breathing with the action of an inhaler, such as children and the elderly.

> ## When to seek help.
> Call your nurse information service or doctor if:
> - Symptoms do not improve after 2 bronchodilator doses.
> - Symptoms increase in frequency or severity.
> - The attack is severe.
> - Your peak-flow meter reading is less than 60% of normal or continues to drop after medication.

CANCER PAIN

What is cancer pain?

Chronic *cancer* pain is discomfort caused by the disease or its treatment. Cancer pain ranges in intensity from mild to severe and takes different forms: dull or sharp, constant or intermittent, throbbing or steady. Not every case of cancer inevitably results in pain; generally, though, the more advanced the cancer, the higher the likelihood of having pain.

Cancer pain can almost always be effectively treated. People with pain from cancer have the right to insist on receiving treatment for it.

What causes cancer pain?

In about 4 out of 5 cases, pain arises from a *tumor* that grows large enough to press on nerves or the spinal cord, or from cancerous cells that invade bones, organs, or blood vessels. Other possible causes include immune system activity; side effects of surgery, radiation, or *chemotherapy*; or indirect effects of the disease, such as infections. Stress, anxiety, and depression (*see* page 238) related to having cancer can make the perception of pain worse.

How is cancer pain treated?

There are several methods of relieving cancer pain. The choice depends on the type, source, and severity of pain and on your own individual needs and circumstances. The more accurately you can describe your pain, the better your caregivers will be able to help you find relief.

Treatment for cancer—for example, surgical removal of a tumor that is pressing on a nerve—is enough, in many cases, to eliminate most or all of the pain.

Medications are also an important aspect of chronic cancer pain treatment. The modern approach involves starting with analgesics (pain relievers) and adding more potent medications as needed. The first step is to start with over-the-counter nonnarcotic products, such as aspirin, acetaminophen, or ibuprofen (*see* page 27). These everyday products are surprisingly effective in managing mild to moderate cancer pain.

If additional relief is needed, the doctor may prescribe higher doses of these medications or add a narcotic medication, such as codeine or morphine. Aspirin plus codeine is a commonly used combination. Most people with severe pain from terminal cancer feel relief from meperidine (e.g., Demerol), morphine, methadone, or other opiate drugs. There is a risk that such treatments may cause sleepiness, confusion, or delirium. Pain arising from cancer that has spread to the bone may be treated with hormones, radio-pharmaceuticals, or X-ray therapy for isolated bone involvement. Other treatments for cancer pain include:

Alternative treatments. Electrostimulation uses electricity to stimulate nerves and disrupt the flow of pain signals to the brain. Acupuncture uses needles to achieve the same goal and may work for some people. In some cases, neurosurgery is performed to sever selected nerves and disrupt the pain signals to the brain. Drugs injected directly into or near to a nerve produce similar effects. While these nerve-blocking strategies are still considered experimental, they are being used more often.

Behavior modification techniques. Biofeedback, hypnosis, relaxation, and cognitive control (through guided imagery or distraction) may have some value for people who experience mild to moderate pain. Part of the benefit of these techniques comes from their ability to decrease anxiety and build confidence in coping with pain. Often these techniques work best as supplemental therapy, in conjunction with medications, in cases of mild pain.

Adjunctive therapy. This treatment for cancer-related complications aims at improving your overall sense of well-being. For example, treatment with antibiotics may clear up a painful infection, while use of an antidepressant medication may relieve the emotional suffering that often accompanies the struggle against a chronic life-threatening illness. Low doses of some types of antidepressants also have pain-relieving properties. Corticosteroids improve mood, reduce swelling and inflammation, and help restore appetite. Sometimes tranquilizers are prescribed to relieve anxiety and discomfort associated with cancer and its treatment. Changing the dose of the drug, the timing of the dose, or the way in which you take it (e.g., by mouth, injection, patch, or suppository) may result in greater pain relief.

Do narcotics pose a risk of addiction?

In the past, some physicians were hesitant to give narcotics out of fear that some patients might become addicted. Such a fear adds unnecessarily to the suffering cancer can cause. Psychological addiction means continued use of a drug after the medical need for it has stopped, or use of the drug merely to experience its effects (to get "high"). Physiological (i.e., physical) addiction means that there is a tolerance built up to the pain-relieving effect of the drug and withdrawal symptoms on stopping the drug. Today, however, pain relief is recognized as a priority in cancer treatment. The proper use of these drugs by people with cancer-related pain—taken when needed in adequate doses—poses little or no risk of addiction, and the benefits far outweigh any potential risk.

When to seek help.

Call your nurse information service or doctor if:

- Your cancer-related pain returns or gets worse.

CATARACT/GLAUCOMA

What is a cataract?

A cataract is an eye defect in which part of the lens, which is normally clear and translucent, becomes cloudy. Cataracts can occur in either or both eyes, causing vision to grow more blurry, usually over a period of years.

What is glaucoma?

Glaucoma is an eye disorder involving an increase of pressure from the aqueous humor (i.e., the fluid between the *cornea* and the iris) that builds up between the cornea of the eye and the lens. This pressure, in turn, causes pressure on the vitreous humor (i.e., the fluid inside the eyeball), which can damage the optic nerve, causing severe vision loss or blindness (*see* figure, page 86). Chronic (i.e., open-angle) glaucoma, which accounts for 9 out of 10 cases, develops over many years. Acute (i.e., closed-angle) glaucoma occurs suddenly and leads to pain and vision loss within a few days.

What causes cataracts and glaucoma?

Cataracts develop after years of exposure to radiation, including *ultraviolet* rays from the sun, X rays, or microwaves. Some cataracts are caused or worsened by eye injury or infections; they can also result from other illnesses, such as diabetes (*see* page 240). Other risk factors include drugs (e.g., steroids), alcohol, and smoking. People may inherit a tendency to develop cataracts.

Glaucoma develops when a drainage network inside the eye becomes clogged, thus preventing the fluid from flowing normally out of the eye. The cause of the blockage is not known. Glaucoma is more prevalent in people of African descent, people with heart disease (*see* page 236), diabetes (*see* page 240), or nearsightedness, and it is more likely to occur in people with a family history of the condition.

What are the symptoms of cataracts and glaucoma?

The main symptom of cataracts is a painless but gradually increasing blurriness of vision or "double vision" (i.e., seeing overlapping images). Often halos (i.e., fuzzy rings) appear around lights. Driving at night may be difficult due to the glare of oncoming headlights. People with cataracts typically become less able to perceive colors, and they may need to change their eyeglass prescriptions frequently. Some people even experience "second sight" (i.e., an improvement in vision) such that they can read without glasses. They may be more sensitive to bright light, and their vision may improve in dim light. As the cataract becomes more severe, the lens may become milky gray or yellow in color.

Chronic glaucoma may not cause any symptoms at first. Gradually, a person may notice loss of peripheral vision or have blind spots. Acute glaucoma produces sudden and severe eye pain, blurred vision, and halos around lights, often accompanied by nausea and vomiting. Without prompt medical attention, blindness may result.

Can cataracts and glaucoma be prevented?

For cataracts, wearing sunglasses that block out the maximum amount of ultraviolet radiation is a sensible precaution. Hats or caps with broad brims or visors can help. However, cataracts are the product of a lifetime of exposure to radiation, and they develop to some degree in about 3 out of 4 people.

There is no known way to prevent glaucoma, but early detection, through regular eye examinations, can reduce the risks.

How are cataracts treated?

If the problem seriously disrupts normal activities, surgery can be done to replace the lens with an artificial implant. The procedure is painless and effective, resulting in dramatically improved vision about 95% of the time. Until surgery is required, ways to cope with cataracts include avoiding bright sunlight, wearing sunglasses with yellow lenses, and using incandescent floor or desk lamps, rather than ceiling fixtures or lamps with halogen bulbs. Large-print books and newspapers are widely available, as are many household products designed to assist the visually impaired with everyday tasks.

How is glaucoma treated?

Treatment for acute glaucoma is aimed at reducing pressure through the regular use of eyedrops. There are 3 main types of drops: miotics cause the pupil to constrict, thus permitting easier drainage of the aqueous humor; adrenergic agonists act on nerves and tissues to promote fluid outflow; beta-blockers, the most common treatment, work by reducing the amount of fluid produced by the eye. A new class of drops called prostaglandins which also lower pressure has just been introduced. If the optic nerve has been damaged or is threatened, treatment includes oral doses of drugs known as carbonic anhydrase inhibitors

(also available as eyedrops). Regular, frequent eye exams are needed to monitor the effectiveness of treatment and to evaluate the extent of nerve damage. Surgery is an option if other treatments fail or you have another condition that prevents use of medication. You may need the surgery more than once.

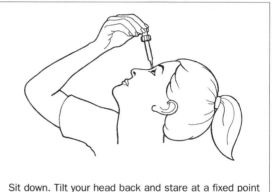

Sit down. Tilt your head back and stare at a fixed point on the ceiling. Keep your eyes wide open. Hold the dropper straight above your eye; do not tilt it. Keep your focus on the ceiling while you use the dropper.

When to seek help.

Seek emergency help if:

- You experience severe eye pain.

- You experience sudden loss of vision in one or both eyes.

Call your nurse information service or doctor if:

- You notice blurry vision, double vision, halos around lights, or sensitivity to light.

- You experience side effects from your glaucoma medication.

CHRONIC BRONCHITIS/EMPHYSEMA

What are chronic bronchitis and emphysema?

Chronic bronchitis is a lasting, recurring infection or irritation of the lungs. The irritation causes the large and small passageways (the bronchi and the bronchioles) that carry air into the lungs to become inflamed and swollen. The inflamed tubes also secrete large amounts of thick mucus, which cause lung congestion and coughing.

Emphysema involves the alveoli, which are little air sacs at the ends of the bronchioles. The sacs, which resemble tiny clusters of grapes, are elastic. They expand when you inhale, holding the oxygen so it can be picked up by blood cells and carried throughout the body. During this exchange, the blood cells release carbon dioxide, which is expelled when you exhale. In emphysema, however, the sacs lose their elasticity; eventually many of them rupture, making breathing—especially exhaling—very difficult. Emphysema also causes the bronchioles to become narrow, further disrupting breathing and trapping stale air inside the lungs.

Chronic bronchitis and emphysema often occur together; these conditions are called chronic obstructive pulmonary disease (COPD).

What causes chronic bronchitis and emphysema?

The most common cause of both diseases is smoking cigarettes or exposure to secondhand tobacco smoke. In rare cases, COPD results from an inherited condition in which the body fails to make a substance called alpha-1-antitrypsin, thus allowing an enzyme to destroy normal airway elasticity. COPD can be an occupational hazard in jobs that require heavy exposure to noxious, irritating fumes. Worsening of chronic bronchitis can be due to an acute viral or bacterial infection. Air pollution or chemical fumes can also cause problems.

What are the symptoms of chronic bronchitis and emphysema?

The symptoms of chronic bronchitis can include shortness of breath, wheezing, difficulty exhaling, and a cough (worse in the morning) that produces large amounts of mucus and that is usually present for 3 months for at least 2 consecutive years. Emphysema also causes shortness of breath, especially on exertion (such as climbing stairs), but the cough is less severe and is "dry" (does not generate mucus).

In severe COPD, coughing may bring up blood and cause persistent chest pain or a bluish complexion, indicating an inadequate oxygen level in your blood. Right-sided heart failure (cor pulmonale) may develop, leading to swollen legs or ankles. People with severe COPD may have a characteristic "barrel-shaped" chest. Damage to the lungs can become progressively worse, eventually leading to dependency on external oxygen sources and death.

How can chronic bronchitis and emphysema be prevented?

The most effective measure is to not smoke cigarettes (for more information on how to stop, *see* page 24). If you have COPD, avoid exposure to smoke, fumes, air pollution, or substances that trigger respiratory allergies (i.e., dust and dust mites, pollen, mold, dander from animals with fur or feathers, chemical fumes, pollution, food additives, and certain medications). Take preventative measures to avoid contracting colds (e.g., wash your hands frequently and avoid contact with sick people) or other respiratory ailments, since these can trigger episodes of bronchitis. Physicians often recommend preventative or immediate use of antibiotics to reduce the risk of infections. If your doctor recomends it, get vaccinated against the flu 6 weeks before the start of each flu season and get a pneumococcal pneumonia vaccination. Some people benefit by changing jobs or moving to a cleaner, warmer, drier climate.

How are chronic bronchitis and emphysema treated?

There is no cure for these illnesses. Treatment is aimed at preventing infections or relieving symptoms.

If you smoke, you must stop! Drinking 8 to 10 glasses of fluids a day thins the mucus and makes it easier to expel; the drug acetylcysteine may also thin secretions. Postural drainage—leaning over and coughing while someone pounds gently on your back—loosens mucus. Adequate humidity keeps air passages moist; use a cool-mist vaporizer or take a hot shower to thin the mucus and make it easier to cough up. Exercise improves breathing capacity, especially walking 5 to 15 minutes, 3 times a day. Breathing exercises may be of value in some cases. Don't use cough suppressants or sedatives.

Inhaled medications, called bronchodilators, relax airway muscles to allow freer breathing. Some physicians recommend use of inhaled corticosteroids (such as beclomethasone) to reduce inflammation, but the value of these drugs in treating COPD is unproved and they are much less effective than in treating asthma. Antibiotics combat bacterial infections but not viral ones. They are generally given at the first sign of a respiratory infection. In severe emergencies, hospitalization may be needed to deliver antibiotics intravenously. People whose bodies lack alpha-1-antitrypsin may benefit from infusions of the missing enzyme.

If your case is severe, you may need continuous, around-the-clock oxygen therapy to boost oxygen levels. Use of diuretics can remove excess fluids from the body, thus relieving the load on the heart. Digitalis is sometimes helpful to treat co-existing heart failure. In extreme cases, you may need a lung transplant or a heart-lung transplant may be necessary.

When to seek help.

If you have a diagnosis of COPD, call your nurse information service or doctor if:

- You develop fever, chest pain, or swelling in the legs or ankles.

- Shortness of breath develops when you are resting or doing minimal physical exercise.

- Your *sputum* is thicker or has blood in it.

- Your complexion turns blue or purple.

CONGESTIVE HEART FAILURE

What is congestive heart failure?

Congestive heart failure (CHF) is a serious, potentially life-threatening condition in which the heart loses its ability to pump effectively. Blood returning to the heart is not pumped through at the proper rate or amount, so it backs up in the lungs and other tissues, causing congestion. Pressure causes fluid to seep out of blood vessels into nearby tissues and blood flow throughout the body slows down. Lack of adequate blood supply in turn interferes with the way various tissues and organs function. At the same time, the heart works harder (i.e., beating faster or irregularly) to compensate for the inadequate oxygen supply. CHF is a progressive condition—it gets worse over time.

What causes CHF?

CHF is primarily a consequence of another disease or physical problem. It begins most often following a heart attack (*see* page 236). Some cases arise from *myocarditis*, or a cardiac defect present since birth. A problem with valves that regulate the flow of blood within the heart's chambers may also be a cause. Other potential risk factors include chronic high blood pressure (*see* page 244); emphysema (*see* page 232); long-standing, untreated hyperthyroidism (*see* page 192); anemia (*see* page 92); or severe nutritional deficiencies. CHF arising on one side of the heart (usually the left) can often lead to CHF on the opposite side.

What are the symptoms of CHF?

When failure occurs on the left side of the heart, blood backs up into the lungs, causing them to become congested with fluid, displacing air and leading to breathlessness, especially on exertion or when lying flat in bed. Some people experience a dry cough or a cough that brings up blood. CHF increases the risk of lung infections, such as *pneumonia*.

Right-sided heart failure makes blood back up into the liver (causing it to enlarge) and legs, leading to edema (*see* page 213) in the lower limbs and ankles. Other symptoms include frequent urination, especially at night; weight gain; abdominal pain and loss of appetite; and swollen neck veins.

In many cases, CHF involves both the left and the right sides. Weakness and fatigue occur when the muscles become starved for blood and oxygen. Other symptoms include *arrhythmia*; low blood pressure; and a sense of anxiety, irritability, restlessness, and, in severe cases or in the elderly, mental confusion.

How can CHF be prevented?

Smoking is a major factor in diseases of the lung and heart, including CHF. Stopping smoking, even after many years, can reduce your risk (*see* page 24). Excess body weight makes the heart work harder; losing weight can help to lighten the load (*see* page 25), as can a diet low in salt and saturated fat (*see* page 17). Avoid overuse of alcohol (*see* page 16), which interferes with heart function. Aerobic exercise helps to condition and maintain the heart (*see* page 20). If you have high blood pressure (*see* page 244), this must be controlled. In cases where another underlying condition is the cause, improved management of the condition can prevent CHF.

How is CHF treated?

Medical treatment options include the use of drugs called diuretics, which increase urination and help speed the elimination of excess fluid, and ACE inhibitors such as captopril, which expand blood vessels, increase blood flow, and reduce blood pressure. Digitalis drugs, such as digoxin, slow the heart rate and improve the heart's ability to contract and, thus, to push blood through the body. Anticoagulants, such as warfarin, are sometimes given to bedridden patients to reduce the risk of blood clots. Other medications can improve blood flow, ease breathing, or reduce anxiety.

People with CHF need to cut back on strenuous physical activities and get plenty of rest. There is a danger that the body's muscles will weaken too much from disuse, however, so your doctor may recommend mild activity (e.g., walking or cycling) or physical therapy. Sleeping with the head elevated (or sleeping sitting up) reduces the risk of lung congestion. Frequently changing leg positions when sitting helps the circulation and prevents swelling or clotting.

Since salt in the diet causes the body to retain excess fluid, cutting down on salt and reducing fluid intake may reduce swelling. Caffeine stimulates the heart, so avoid consuming too many caffeinated beverages and foods (e.g., coffee, tea, cola, or chocolate). Eating smaller, more frequent meals can facilitate digestion and lower the load on the heart. Wearing support stockings applies pressure to the vessels in the legs and reduces swelling.

In severe CHF, some people may need oxygen therapy to help them breathe. Surgery may be needed to repair or replace damaged heart valves or replace or widen blocked arteries. Heart transplants are sometimes required.

When to seek help.

Seek emergency help if:

- You experience severe breathlessness.
- You have severe chest pain.

Call your nurse information service or doctor if:

- You are being treated for CHF and you develop a fever, or your symptoms, including breathlessness and rapid or irregular heartbeat, get worse.
- You develop any of the following symptoms: dizziness, blurred vision, dry cough that won't go away, increased fatigue, decreased urine output, or weight increase of 3 to 5 pounds in one week.

CORONARY HEART DISEASE

What is coronary heart disease (CHD)?

Coronary *arteries* are vessels on the surface of the heart that carry blood to the heart muscle. Over time, *plaque* can build up inside these arteries, causing them to become stiff and narrow and reducing the amount of blood that flows through them. This process, atherosclerosis, is sometimes called "hardening of the arteries." Ischemia (i.e., reduced blood supply) deprives the heart muscle of the oxygen and nutrients it needs to function. Sometimes blood clots form in the narrowed arteries, stopping blood flow completely.

What happens if the heart doesn't get enough blood?

When arteries in the body narrow, this leads to high blood pressure (*see* page 244). The heart has to work harder to pump blood.

Further serious consequences of CHD are angina and myocardial infarction (MI) (i.e., heart attack). Symptoms of angina include pain, usually in the chest, and a feeling of burning, pressure, or tightness. There may be associated shortness of breath or *palpitations*. The pain may seem to be in the shoulders or arms. Symptoms, which last a few minutes, usually get better with rest or drugs, such as nitroglycerin. Sometimes, however, there are no symptoms; this is called silent ischemia. Angina, especially if it occurs during rest, becomes more severe, or begins to last longer, is often a warning sign that a heart attack may occur in the future.

Heart attack results when the artery becomes completely blocked, usually by plaque or a blood clot. Sudden loss of blood supply results in severe, often permanent or fatal damage to the heart muscle. Heart attacks frequently occur without warning or symptoms (i.e., silent MI). Pain can be excruciating, lasting 30 minutes or more, and it does not go away with rest or nitroglycerin.

Can anything prevent CHD?

Some risk factors for CHD are beyond your control, including advanced age, being male, or having a family history of heart disease. Changing your lifestyle, however, can help control angina and prevent heart attacks or recurrences.

Stop smoking. If you have heart disease, it's very important to stop smoking (*see* page 24). Talk with your doctor about which strategy is right for you.

Watch your diet. The fatty deposits in arteries include cholesterol. Reducing saturated fat and cholesterol in your diet may minimize plaque buildup. Also, decreasing the amount of salt in your diet may reduce arterial stiffness (*see* page 17).

Lose weight. People whose body weight is 30% higher than average have a greater risk of CHD. Losing weight through a sensible program of balanced nutrition (*see* page 17) and exercise (*see* page 20) can help reduce the load on your heart.

Exercise. Inactivity is a big risk factor for CHD. Exercising, regardless of your age, can lessen arterial stiffness and reduce your danger of CHD (*see* page 20). Before undertaking any weight loss or exercise program, talk with your doctor.

Keep blood pressure low. The above strategies also help lower blood pressure, which in turn reduces risk of CHD. In addition, your doctor may prescribe medication to lower blood pressure.

Monitor diabetes (*see* page 240). Diet, exercise, and weight loss will help control your blood sugar if you have diabetes. Medications may also be necessary.

Educate yourself. Know the warning signs of heart attack:

- Uncomfortable pressure, fullness, squeezing, or pain in the chest lasting longer than 2 minutes.
- Pain spreading to the shoulders, arms, or neck.
- Dizziness, fainting, sweating, nausea, or shortness of breath.

How is CHD treated?

Medication is usually the first choice of treatment for angina. Drugs can improve blood flow through the arteries or reduce the heart's workload. Options include nitroglycerin, beta blockers, and calcium channel blockers, which may lower the risk of arterial *spasms* and control irregular heartbeats. Aspirin (*see* page 27) can prevent blood clots; check with your doctor before taking aspirin for this purpose. Vitamin E may be of some benefit, but this is unproven. When a heart attack occurs, thrombolytic drugs can be given to dissolve blood clots quickly.

Surgery can be both treatment for heart attacks and an option to prevent angina and heart attacks. Angioplasty is a technique for widening arteries by inflating a balloon inside the artery to flatten the layer of plaque or by using a special scraping tool to cut away the plaque. Another approach is coronary artery bypass, in which a length of vein is removed from elsewhere in the body

and sewn into the coronary artery to bypass the blocked area.

When to seek help.

Seek emergency help if:

- You think you are having a heart attack. Don't assume the pain will subside. Medications can be given to dissolve blood clots and, thus, prevent a heart attack from progressing, reducing the risk of permanent damage or death.

Call your nurse information service or doctor if:

- You have unexplained chest pain that lasts for more than a few minutes.

DEPRESSION

What is depression?

Depression is a serious mental illness involving deep feelings of sadness and despair. Everyone feels sad or "blue" at times, but depression lasts for weeks, even months, causing difficulty in thinking, producing physical symptoms, and profoundly disrupting life, activities, and relationships. One out of 10 people will experience depression at some time.

There are several types of depression. Major depression involves one or more periods of deep sadness, followed by a return to normal functioning. Dysthymia causes low moods that are less severe but that last for 2 years or more. Bipolar disorder (i.e., "manic depression") involves dramatic mood swings, from intense highs to profound lows. Seasonal affective disorder occurs in winter and is triggered by reduced sunlight during the day.

What causes depression?

Depression is a physical as well as a mental illness. This is important, because people with depression are not able to just "cheer up" or "snap out of it." Depression arises from a number of factors. Because the illness runs in families, some people may be prone to depression. Neurotransmitters (i.e., brain chemicals) regulate moods, and problems with these chemicals can produce depression. Often depression arises following a specific life event, such as the death of a loved one, childbirth, divorce, or menopause (*see* page 206).

Some depressions arise from misuse of alcohol or illicit drugs, especially marijuana and cocaine. Certain prescription medications, such as tranquilizers or drugs for high blood pressure (*see* page 240), can cause depression as a side effect. Depression can also emerge after a serious disease, such as *pneumonia* or heart attack (*see* page 236).

What are the symptoms of depression?

Major symptoms of depression include feelings of deep sadness, hopelessness, helplessness, guilt, and a sense of worthlessness. People with depression often feel tired, anxious, and irritable. Their speech and movements slow down. They lose interest in things they formerly enjoyed, including socializing, hobbies, and sex. They experience difficulties with thinking, concentrating, and remembering. They withdraw from family and friends and have trouble at work or school. Focusing on the negative, they are prone to suicidal thinking or behavior. Perhaps 15% of suicides are related to depression.

Physical complaints include aches and pains, headaches, agitation, and constipation. Some depressed people can barely drag themselves out of bed. Others wake early in the morning and are unable to fall back to sleep. Some people lose their appetite and lose weight, while others overeat and gain weight.

Major depression lasts for at least 2 weeks, and the symptoms may fluctuate in severity during the day. People may have only one episode of major depression, or they may suffer a number of episodes over time. Dysthymia causes more "down days" than "up days" for at least 2 years. The manic phase of bipolar disorder lasts at least a week and is followed by the "crash" of the depressive phase. Seasonal affective disorder begins in the fall and lasts until spring.

How can depression be prevented?

Remain active. Regular physical activity, such as exercise, prevents depression and reduces symptoms. Hobbies, vacations, and socializing can all help to keep depression at bay. Turn off the TV, and engage in more stimulating activities.

Avoid mood-altering drugs. Don't use illicit drugs (*see* page 19) or alcohol, which is a depressant (*see* page 16). Use prescription drugs only as directed. If you smoke, try to quit (*see* page 24). Learn a relaxation technique, such as yoga or meditation (*see* page 23).

Talk to someone. Speak to a trusted friend, relative, or counselor (e.g., a pastor).

Read about depression. Educate yourself about the illness and learn healthier ways of thinking.

How is depression treated?

Most people get better with a combination of psychotherapy and medication. In private, group, or family sessions with a psychologist or a psychiatrist, you can explore life issues and find ways to change your emotional and behavioral responses.

There are several types of antidepressants available; if one type doesn't work, another may. Today the drugs most widely prescribed are those that regulate the brain chemical serotonin. These drugs (e.g., Prozac) work as well or better than the older antidepressants (i.e., tricyclics, such as imipramine) and cause fewer side effects. Monoamine oxidase inhibitors (MAOIs) are also effective but may have serious side effects; people taking these need to avoid certain foods, such as

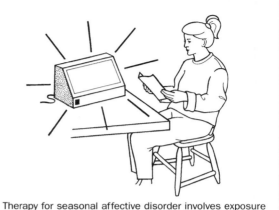

Therapy for seasonal affective disorder involves exposure to bright light to reset the body's biological clock and may include the use of a light box.

cheese. New drugs regularly appear on the market.

Manic depression requires prolonged treatment with medication, generally lithium. For severe depression that does not respond to other treatments, hospitalization and electroconvulsive therapy (ECT) may be needed.

Take antidepressants as directed even if you are not currently feeling depressed. Depression can return even after a lapse of years.

When to seek help.

Call your nurse information service or doctor if:

- You have thoughts of suicide.
- Your depression progressively worsens.
- Your depression interferes with work or family activity.

DIABETES

What is diabetes?

Your body transforms some of the food you eat into glucose, a sugar that supplies cells with energy. Normally, glucose travels in the blood and enters cells with the help of insulin, a hormone produced by the pancreas. Diabetes is a condition in which glucose cannot enter cells because of an insulin problem, resulting in dangerously high blood glucose levels. There is no cure for diabetes, but you can live an otherwise normal, active life if you carefully monitor and control glucose levels every day, plan meals, exercise, maintain a normal body weight (*see* page 25), and take medications as prescribed.

What are the risks of diabetes?

Diabetes can cause acids to build up in the blood (ketoacidosis) and along with very high blood sugars can lead to nausea/vomiting, fatigue, unquenchable thirst, coma, and even death. Over time, diabetes can cause poor circulation, with damage to the feet and legs that can lead to amputation, severe nerve damage, kidney disease, heart disease (*see* page 236), stroke (*see* page 156), eye disease, blindness, or death. If glucose levels fall too low, *hypoglycemia* may occur, causing trembling, weakness, sweating, palpitations, fatigue, dizziness, and possibly coma.

How is diabetes treated?

There are 2 main types of diabetes. Although they are managed differently, the goal is the same: to control glucose levels and prevent complications.

Insulin-dependent diabetes (IDD or Type I) arises when the pancreas does not produce insulin.

People with IDD must take insulin injections every day to survive. Type I diabetes generally begins in people under 20 years of age.

Noninsulin-dependent diabetes (NIDD or Type II) is more common and occurs when the body's insulin does not function properly. Many people with NIDD can control the disease through diet and exercise alone. Others require oral drugs or injected insulin. Type II diabetes often runs in families.

Treatment plan. Your health-care providers will design a diabetes care plan tailored to your needs. It is your responsibility to carry out that plan daily and make essential lifestyle changes. Keep all medical appointments, including those for blood and eye tests.

Self-monitoring of glucose. The goal is to attain good control over blood glucose levels or to keep the levels as close to normal as possible. Research has shown that good glucose control dramatically lowers the risk of developing complications. Your health-care providers will determine what level is normal for you and will teach you how and when to measure levels. You may need to monitor from 1 to 4 times daily, depending on your type of diabetes. Extra testing may be required if your diet or exercise plan changes, if you travel, if you have an acute illness, or if glucose levels are too high or too low. Record your levels in a diary that you can bring with you to medical appointments. Your doctor may also administer a special blood test, called a glycosylated hemoglobin or hemoglobin A1C, to show your average glucose levels over the past 3 to 4 months and indicate how your management plan is working.

Diet. Your health-care providers will help you plan the size, content, and frequency of your meals. Failure to follow this plan carefully increases your risk of excessively high or low glucose levels. Being overweight increases your need for insulin, so controlling or losing weight can help (*see* page 25). Limit fat, sugars, and calories. Eat nutritionally balanced meals (*see* page 17). Avoid high-cholesterol, high-fat, or salty foods to reduce the risk of heart disease (*see* page 236) and high blood pressure (*see* page 244). Limit alcohol consumption (*see* page 16).

Exercise. Physical fitness both strengthens the heart and improves circulation, aids metabolism (i.e., the body's use of food, including glucose), and helps control weight—all important considerations for a person with diabetes. Ask your health-care provider to recommend an exercise program. Generally, a good plan involves aerobic exercise—walking, running, swimming, or cycling—for half an hour 3 to 4 times a week. Eat a snack 30 minutes before exercise, and have carbohydrates available during exercise. To reduce the risk of glucose levels that are too low, avoid exercising at times when insulin injections have their peak effect.

Medication. If you have IDD, you will need to give yourself daily insulin injections. The number of these injections will depend on your condition and the type of insulin prescribed. People with NIDD who can't control glucose levels through diet and exercise take oral (i.e., by mouth) hypoglycemic agents, which increase the body's output (i.e., use) of insulin.

Other steps. Keep snacks with you in case of low blood sugar reactions; try dried fruit or orange juice, and ask your doctor for other snack ideas. Stop smoking (*see* page 24). Take good care of your feet. Have regular eye and physician exams. Make sure your family understands your condition and how it is being managed. Wear a medical-alert ID bracelet. Follow your doctor's instructions.

When to seek help.

Call your nurse information service or doctor if:

- You have trouble controlling glucose levels.
- You experience complications, such as hypoglycemia, fever, nausea, and vomiting.
- You want to change your care plan.

HIV INFECTION

What is HIV infection?

Infection with HIV (i.e., human immunodeficiency virus) occurs when the virus enters the body and attaches itself to certain white blood cells (i.e., T lymph cells), which are essential parts of the immune system. The virus penetrates the cells and begins to reproduce, killing the T cells. As the immune system breaks down, the body becomes vulnerable to other serious diseases. Over time, HIV infection progresses to full-blown AIDS (acquired immune deficiency syndrome).

How is HIV transmitted?

HIV is transmitted via body fluids (e.g., blood, semen, and vaginal secretions) through unprotected sexual contact, exposure to contaminated blood and blood products via transfusions, use of infected hypodermic needles (especially needles shared by users of illegal drugs, such as heroin), and transmission by a mother to a fetus during pregnancy or to an infant through breast milk. HIV does not get transmitted by contact with toilet seats or doorknobs, or by casual contact with infected persons.

What are the symptoms of HIV infection?

In the brief early phase, called primary infection, most people with HIV infection experience a syndrome much like mononucleosis (*see* page 102). The syndrome arises suddenly, lasts 3 to 14 days, and involves symptoms including fever, sweating, lethargy, muscle and joint pain, headaches, sensitivity to light, diarrhea, sore throat, swollen lymph glands, rash on the chest and abdomen, depression, irritability, loss of appetite, weight loss, and pain behind the eyes. However, many people with primary infection experience few or no symptoms. It's important to be tested regularly for HIV, whether you have symptoms or not. Call your nurse information service or doctor and ask how you can get tested.

The second phase begins when the body produces HIV antibodies to fight off the infection. A positive blood test indicates these antibodies are present, thus confirming HIV infection. This phase (known as asymptomatic seropositivity) can last 5 to 10 years or more, during which the person may not experience any symptoms of HIV infection but is still very contagious.

The third phase, known as pre-AIDS or AIDS-related complex (ARC), generally lasts for 3 to 5 years and occurs when the immune system begins to lose the battle against the virus. At this time, many serious but not necessarily life-threatening conditions may develop. Symptoms include persistent swollen lymph glands, fungal infections, *parasitic infections*, vaginal infections in women, a "hairy" growth on the tongue (i.e., hairy leukoplakia), skin problems (e.g., acute onset of psoriasis or severe seborrheic dermatitis [*see* page 66]), herpes infections (*see* page 101), night sweats, weight loss, and diarrhea.

Full-blown AIDS involves severe infections, *cancers*, and various illnesses of the lungs, heart, digestive system, and central nervous system. There is now no known cure, and the disease appears to be fatal (although there are cases of people with HIV who feel well after 15 or more years).

How can HIV infection be prevented?

Always using a latex condom treated with a spermicide helps prevent transmission of the virus between sexual partners but is not foolproof. The virus can enter via tiny wounds in delicate membranes, so unprotected vaginal, oral, or anal sex with infected partners should be avoided. Sex with multiple partners increases risk, but you can also get HIV through a single encounter. Drug users should not share needles and should seek treatment to stop using drugs (*see* page 19).

How is HIV infection treated?

Treatment has three goals: to prevent infections and diseases from developing, to relieve symptoms of medical problems that do occur, and to slow the progression to full-blown AIDS.

Vaccines prevent a range of illnesses to which people with HIV are susceptible, including *hepatitis* B, *tetanus*, and *measles*. People with HIV should avoid oral polio, typhoid, and yellow fever vaccines, because in people with weak immune systems these vaccines may cause the very diseases they are meant to prevent. Use of flu vaccine is controversial. When T cell counts fall to a certain level, therapy is given to prevent some of the more serious, common AIDS-related infections. Strategies include trimethoprim-sulfamethoxazole to prevent toxoplasmosis and pneumocystic pneumonia, and isoniazid for *tuberculosis*.

There are many treatments available to fight the various fungal, bacterial, and viral infections and other diseases that arise in people with HIV. Examples include nystatin or fluconazole for treatment of thrush (i.e., a fungal infection of the mouth and tongue), penicillin for syphilis (*see* page 101), acyclovir for herpes infection (*see* page 101), and radiation therapy or anticancer drugs for Kaposi's sarcoma (a form of skin cancer).

Antiviral drugs interfere with the virus's ability to reproduce, thus slowing the progression to full-blown AIDS. Treatment with zidovudine (ZDV, formerly known as AZT; brand name, Retrovir) or acyclovir that begins soon after exposure to HIV can prolong a person's life. Zidovudine may also help reduce the transmission of HIV from a pregnant woman to her unborn fetus. Other treatments include didanosine (ddI; brand name, Videx) and zalcitabine (ddC). Recently new antiviral agents known as protease inhibitors came on the market. These drugs (the first was saquinivir; brand name, Invirase) cause the virus to reproduce in a form that can't infect new cells. Many other drugs and drug combinations are under study, but there is no vaccine to prevent HIV infection nor any proven treatment that will eliminate the virus. HIV therapy is costly and poses a risk of serious adverse effects, including nausea, diarrhea, headaches, and seizures. Because HIV infection disrupts life on so many levels, people living with the virus often benefit from counseling, social support, and treatment for depression (*see* page 238) or other emotional and psychiatric problems.

When to seek help.

Call your nurse information service or doctor if:

- You may have been exposed to HIV infection through sex with an infected person or by sharing hypodermic needles.
- You experience symptoms of HIV infection.
- You are pregnant and think you may have been exposed to HIV in the past.

HYPERTENSION (HIGH BLOOD PRESSURE)

What is hypertension?

As the heart pumps, pressure forces blood to move through the arteries. Hypertension, or high blood pressure, occurs when the pressure reaches high, unhealthy levels. Left untreated, hypertension can damage blood vessels throughout the body. Risks include *arteriosclerosis*, kidney damage, vision loss, heart attack and heart failure (*see* page 236), and stroke (*see* page 258).

Blood pressure is measured in 2 stages, each of which is given a separate number. Systolic pressure is the force with which the heart pumps blood into the arteries; diastolic pressure is the level present when the heart relaxes and is thus always a lower number. An average healthy blood pressure reading is about 120/80 mm Hg (i.e., millimeters of mercury), but the definition of normal depends on such factors as age, gender, and general health. However, a reading of 140/90 or above is often considered a sign of elevated blood pressure requiring lifestyle changes and/or treatment.

What causes hypertension?

Nine out of 10 cases have no identifiable cause. Doctors refer to this as primary (i.e, essential) hypertension. In other cases, hypertension may result from pregnancy or a medical condition, such as a kidney disorder or hormonal imbalance. Hypertension arising from an underlying cause is known as secondary hypertension.

What are the symptoms of hypertension?

Most people with hypertension notice no symptoms. In severe cases, symptoms may include dizziness, headaches, mental confusion, or nosebleeds.

Can hypertension be prevented?

Getting regular medical checkups is an important part of preventing and detecting hypertension. Blood pressure readings are a part of routine medical examinations. If the levels are high, repeated measurements establish whether the hypertension is persistent or merely temporary. When hypertension is detected early, treatment may be easier and more effective.

Certain risk factors for hypertension cannot be avoided. Risks are higher for males, blacks, and people with a family history of the disorder. However, there are steps you can take to minimize the risk. These include losing weight (*see* page 25), exercising (*see* page 20), changing your diet (e.g., decreasing salt, fat, and cholesterol; increasing calcium and potassium) (*see* page 17), restricting alcohol intake (*see* page 16), avoiding excessive use of decongestants and diet pills, reducing stress, and stopping smoking (*see* page 24).

How is hypertension treated?

Controlling hypertension is a lifetime commitment aimed at preventing the development of serious complications. The first strategy is to make changes in lifestyle, specifically through diet and exercise. In mild cases, cutting back on salt, taking part in a sensible exercise program (i.e., 20 to 30 minutes of vigorous exercise, 3 times a week), losing weight, and learning relaxation techniques may be all the treatment you need. Frequent blood pressure monitoring at home, using special instruments, can help you keep track of your progress. You should monitor your blood pressure several times a week in a resting, non-hurried state and not immediately following a meal. Because hypertension may not cause any symptoms, you need to stick with your treatment plan even if you feel perfectly fine.

If these techniques are ineffective, there are many types of medications (i.e., antihypertensives) that can control primary hypertension. As a rule, once you start taking these drugs, you need to keep taking them for the rest of your life. That's why the best approach is to try lifestyle changes first.

Diuretics ("water pills") are usually the first choice for treatment of hypertension. These drugs speed up the elimination of salt and water from the body, which reduces the volume of the fluid in the blood and causes the small arteries to relax. However, in the process, these drugs can also remove another important substance, potassium, from your body. You may need potassium supplements if you take diuretics. Other antihypertensives work by directly affecting the blood vessels or the nerves that control them:

- Alpha blockers and central alpha agonists block the activity of nerves that cause vessels to constrict.

- Angiotensin-converting-enzyme (ACE) inhibitors prevent the formation of angiotensin, a chemical that triggers blood vessel constriction.

- Beta blockers reduce the activity of heart nerves, causing the heart to beat more slowly and with less force.

- Calcium channel blockers prevent calcium from entering cells in the arterial walls, thus keeping the arteries from narrowing.

- Vasodilators act directly on the arteries, causing them to relax.

Because these drugs act in different ways, doctors sometimes prescribe a combination of 2 or more, often a diuretic and a beta blocker, ACE inhibitor, or calcium channel blocker. If one drug doesn't work or if it causes unacceptable side effects, switching to another drug will often do the job.

In cases of secondary hypertension, treatment aimed at the primary problem (e.g., a kidney disorder) often helps blood pressure return to normal without the need for specific antihypertensive medications.

When to seek help.

Call your nurse information service or doctor if:

- You have high blood pressure and experience dizziness, nosebleeds, confusion, or headaches that last.

- You experience side effects from antihypertensive drugs.

- You checked your blood pressure several times in a given week and the average reading is greater than 140/90, despite lifestyle changes and/or medication.

LOW BACK PAIN

What is low back pain?

Low back pain arises in the "small" of the back—the triangular area above the buttocks. Chronic (i.e., long-lasting) low back pain can range in severity from a dull ache to sharp pain that spreads to other parts of the body.

What causes low back pain?

Low back pain is the result of strained muscles, muscle spasms, or pulled ligaments. Some cases may arise from another ailment, such as arthritis (*see* page 224) or a *prolapsed disk*. Often back pain is caused by stress or injury occurring over a long time: poor posture, extended sitting, vibrations from vehicles or machinery, lack of exercise, poor physical condition, or prolonged tension. Frequently, though, the pain comes on suddenly, as a result of poor lifting techniques, repetitive twisting movements, a fall, or an accident. Even everyday movements, such as intense sneezing or coughing, can trigger pain. Usually such acute (i.e., short-term) injuries heal completely. Back pain often develops for no obvious reason and is called nonspecific backache. There are many causes of back pain, some of which may be serious (e.g., bone infections or *tumors*, aortic *aneurysms*, kidney infections). Unexplained, sudden, or persistent severe back pain or pain with other symptoms (e.g., fever) requires a doctor's evaluation.

What are the symptoms of low back pain?

The main symptom is mild to severe pain in the affected area, appearing suddenly, overnight, or over a period of days. The pain can be constant, or it can appear only when you move a certain way or assume a certain position. Stiffness can develop. Pain and stiffness can be so severe as to make it impossible to move.

How can low back pain be prevented?

The best way to deal with back pain is to prevent it from occurring. Once the back is injured, the risk of reinjury is much higher.

Exercise to keep back, abdominal, and leg muscles in shape. A good strategy is to get at least mild exercise every day and engage in more strenuous activity (e.g., brisk walking, swimming, bicycling, or jogging) for 30 minutes, 3 times a week (*see* page 20).

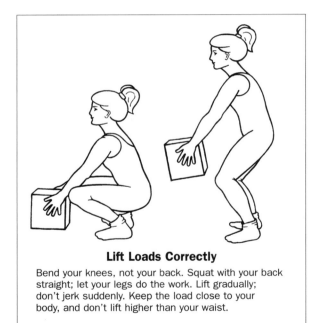

Lift Loads Correctly
Bend your knees, not your back. Squat with your back straight; let your legs do the work. Lift gradually; don't jerk suddenly. Keep the load close to your body, and don't lift higher than your waist.

Maintain good posture. Avoid slouching; keep your head up, shoulders straight, and chest out. Balance weight evenly between the feet when standing. Avoid shoes with high heels or platform soles.

Sit up straight in a firm, high-backed chair. Avoid slumping, and use a pillow if necessary at the base of your spine. Get out of your chair often. When driving, sit close to the wheel so your legs are not fully extended. Stop for frequent rests—get out of the car, then stretch and move around.

Sleep on a firm mattress. If your mattress does not provide adequate support, put a board under it. The best sleep position is on your side, with your knees drawn up slightly. Use a flat pillow for your head. If you sleep on your back, put a pillow under your knees.

Lose weight as your doctor recommends (*see* page 25). Obesity (*see* page 248) strains back muscles.

How is back pain treated?

Almost all cases of sudden back pain heal completely with bed rest and over-the-counter analgesic medications. Depending on the cause or duration of the problem, these strategies may also help relieve chronic pain.

Drugs. Nonsteroidal anti-inflammatory drugs (NSAIDs) (*see* page 28) usually help. Call your doctor if you are being treated or followed for other health problems before taking these products. Most muscle relaxants—actually minor tranquilizers—are no more effective than NSAIDs at relieving pain, but they can promote sleep. Opioid narcotics are seldom needed, except for acute pain during the first or second night of symptoms. Corticosteroid injections can work for limited periods if the pain is confined to a specific spot.

Rest. For the first 24 to 72 hours, lie on a mattress or the floor, with your back flat and legs drawn up. Apply ice for 20 minutes frequently throughout the day. Warm baths after 24 to 48 hours may be

soothing. If the pain lasts, consult your nurse information service or doctor.

Exercises. Try to return to your normal activity level as soon as possible. Ask your doctor about simple floor exercises. Do aerobic exercises gradually over a 2-week period but avoid strengthening exercises that involve back and abdominal muscles. At first, back pain symptoms may recur slightly. If the pain is severe, do different exercises.

Physical therapy. Gentle massages, special exercises, or the use of corsets, braces, or traction help some people; long-term use of braces, however, can lead to muscle weakness and can be counterproductive. Shoe insoles may help people who must stand for long periods.

Chiropractic care. A visit to a chiropractor can sometimes be helpful.

Surgery. Operations are needed in less than 1% of cases of back pain.

When to seek help.

Call your nurse information service or doctor if:

- Pain is severe or lasts for 3 to 4 days.
- Your back pain is due to a fall or injury.
- Pain, weakness, or numbness develops in your legs or feet.
- You have symptoms such as painful urination, flu, gastrointestinal distress, abdominal pain, or fever.
- You lose bladder or bowel control.

OBESITY

What is obesity?

Obesity is excess body weight that is severe enough to pose a threat to health. Being a few pounds overweight is not the same thing as being obese. While not exactly a disease, obesity—especially involving excess weight in the upper body—is a risk factor for a number of other potentially life-endangering medical problems, ranging from diabetes (*see* page 240), kidney disease, and *cancer*, to high blood pressure (*see* page 244), heart disease (*see* page 236), and stroke (*see* page 258).

What causes obesity?

The main cause of obesity is excess intake of calories that is not balanced by an equal expenditure of energy. If you eat too much food and don't burn enough calories, you'll gain excess body weight. This can also happen if you eat relatively normal amounts but get too little exercise. Usually the problem is purely behavioral, involving poor eating and exercise habits, or it may reflect an underlying psychiatric problem, such as depression (*see* page 238) or an eating disorder.

Research shows that some cases of obesity may have a genetic cause. Some people gain weight because their bodies have a lower *metabolism*—in other words, they need fewer calories to function, so they gain weight even if they eat normal quantities of food. A small fraction of cases may involve genetic defects, hormonal imbalances or dysfunctions, or other physical causes.

What are the symptoms of obesity?

Medically speaking, obesity is defined as body weight at more than 20% higher than the upper limits of the recommended level for a person's height and body type (*see* figures, page 26). It is more a function of percentage of body fat content than just weight. Symptoms of obesity can include shortness of breath; low back pain; leg, knee, and foot pain; heartburn; and depression.

Can obesity be prevented?

In many cases, yes. Eat a healthy, balanced diet (*see* page 17). Maintain good eating habits: Establish regular mealtimes, limit snacks, and go easy on desserts and second helpings. Eat slowly, especially when hungry, and stop eating when your hunger is satisfied. The other important aspect in weight control is exercise (*see* page 20), which helps burn off unwanted calories and improves calorie utilization by increasing muscle mass. It's important that the exercise plan be one that you can stick with for a long time.

How is obesity treated?

Many people with obesity are so eager to lose weight that they will follow any fad diet or "miracle" program. While they may lose some pounds and keep them off for a while, almost inevitably the weight returns. This "yo-yo dieting" causes enormous frustration and disappointment and can even lead to an overall increase of body weight and other health problems, such as vitamin deficiencies. A more effective method is to talk to health-care professionals (e.g., a physician, nurse, dietitian, nutritionist, or exercise therapist) and develop a complete strategy aimed at making permanent lifestyle changes.

To promote weight loss, many medically oriented programs recommend a daily intake of 1,200 calories (2,000 to 2,500 calories per day is a standard diet), but this amount will vary with a person's age, gender, size, and overall medical condition. Such a diet emphasizes low-fat, low-caloric foods; avoids animal fats and other saturated fats; and provides a good balance of proteins, carbohydrates, and unsaturated fats. More important than the number of calories is the balance between intake and expenditure. If you burn off 750 more calories each day than you take in, you can lose about 1.5 pounds a week.

The second critical component of an obesity management plan is regular exercise. A typical plan calls for vigorous exercise 30 minutes or more a day, 3 or more times a week. The type of exercise you do is less important than the fact that you are doing it. Some people might prefer biking; others would rather swim. Find an exercise routine that you enjoy and can continue doing indefinitely. Many people find it easier to stick with the plan if they exercise with a friend.

Some people have taken extreme steps such as wiring the jaw shut to prevent eating or stapling the stomach to make it hold less food. Many people have undergone liposuction (i.e., the surgical removal of fat). These procedures pose some risks and will not produce the desired results of permanent weight reduction.

Some individuals may benefit from psychiatric treatments or psychological therapy to address emotional problems and issues that center on food. Patient groups, such as Overeaters Anonymous, can provide insight, strategies, and emotional support.

Appetite-suppressant drugs like phentermine are used for short-term weight loss. In 1996, new drug treatments for morbid obesity (i.e., unhealthy or disease-causing) were approved by the U.S. Food and Drug Administration. These products, including fenfluramine (i.e., Pondimin) and dexfenfluramine (i.e., Redux) are intended for use by severely overweight individuals. As of this writing, it is too soon to know how effective these 2 drugs will be or what side effects are likely to occur. They should only be administered under the supervision of a physician.

If your child is gaining weight more rapidly than standard growth charts suggest is normal, try the following: If your baby is not hungry, do not force her to eat (e.g., do not encourage her to finish her bottle if she's not interested); reduce your child's intake of sweet or fatty food and substitute unsweetened fruits and vegetables; give your child well-diluted, unsweetened fruit drinks and, if she's over 2 years old, low-fat or nonfat milk; and encourage her to be physically active.

> ## When to seek help.
> Call your nurse information service or doctor if:
>
> - You are significantly overweight and have tried to lose weight but have been unsuccessful.
> - You want to improve your diet, change eating habits, or develop an exercise program.

OSTEOPOROSIS

What is osteoporosis?

Osteoporosis is a condition involving gradual loss of the minerals in bones. Over time, the bones lose part of their mass and become porous, weak, and highly vulnerable to breaks or *fractures*. The bones most commonly affected are those in the spine, hips, and wrists. Osteoporosis is a normal condition of aging, affecting 4 times as many women as men. In severe cases, osteoporosis leads to pain, suffering, and disability, due primarily to the loss of mobility and the subsequent health risks following a bone fracture.

What causes osteoporosis?

Like other tissues, the cells and structures in the bones are constantly being renewed. As minerals, such as phosphorus and calcium, dissolve and are removed, the body brings in a new supply to replace what has been lost. With age, however, the rate of loss exceeds the body's ability to replenish the minerals. Bones, once solid and sturdy, become brittle and full of empty spaces.

In osteoporosis, the imbalance between bone buildup and breakdown is accelerated by hormonal changes, especially (in women) the loss of estrogen following menopause (*see* page 206). Insufficient calcium in the diet (especially during adolescence when there is rapid bone growth) is an important factor, since without an adequate supply of calcium, the body can't maintain bone integrity. Exercise inhibits calcium loss and may stimulate bone growth; conversely, lack of exercise can accelerate bone loss. Other risk factors include smoking; drinking alcohol; being underweight; having certain medical conditions, such as hormonal imbalances or chronic lung diseases; using corticosteroids or thyroid replacement hormones for long periods of time; and long periods of bed rest.

What are the symptoms of osteoporosis?

Osteoporosis usually causes no symptoms until far advanced. Pain then develops in certain bones, especially in the lower back. Loss of bone mass causes some bones to become compressed, leading to loss of height and "dowager's hump" (i.e., increasingly stooped posture). Affected bones, especially in the wrist, hips, or spine, are more likely to break or fracture following relatively minor trauma. Osteoporosis will not show up on X ray until about 30% of the bone (calcium) has been lost.

Can osteoporosis be prevented?

The sooner you take steps to prevent osteoporosis, the more effective those steps will be in the long run. Getting adequate calcium through diet or supplements is an important preventative measure. For people at risk, a daily calcium intake of 1,000 to 1,500 milligrams is usually recommended. You may need supplements to reach that level. The main calcium-rich foods are dairy products, but there is some calcium in leafy green vegetables, beans, nuts, fortified orange juice, and cereals. It's also

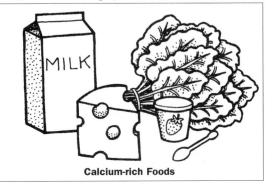

Calcium-rich Foods

important to get adequate vitamin D (about 400 IU/day), which helps the body absorb and use calcium, and 15 to 20 minutes of direct sun exposure per day.

Exercise can also help keep bones strong (*see* page 20). However, the exercise must be regular and "weight-bearing." For example, jogging or walking build bone more efficiently than swimming. Other weight-bearing exercise includes tennis, cycling, dancing, skiing, low-impact aerobics, and weight training. The risk of osteoporosis is higher in smokers, so it's critical to stop smoking (*see* page 24).

Many women benefit from starting long-term *estrogen replacement therapy (ERT)* as soon as possible after menopause. Although they may still lose some bone, the rate of loss will be slower. ERT does not replace lost bone, and bone loss develops rapidly if ERT is stopped. Not all women are eligible for ERT, and there is some risk of adverse effects. The pros and cons of ERT vary with each individual, so you should discuss them fully with a member of your health care team.

How is osteoporosis treated?

Once osteoporosis develops, treatment is designed to slow down any further loss of bone minerals, restore as much bone mass as possible, and prevent fractures. The most basic step involves increased intake of calcium and vitamin D through diet and supplements.

ERT is the standard treatment for women who develop osteoporosis after menopause and who do not have breast *cancer* or a strong family history of breast cancer. ERT works by slowing bone mineral loss, and is available in oral doses or as a skin patch. For women who are not eligible for ERT, calcium supplements (1500 mg/day) and vitamin D (400 IU/day) are the best strategy. Drugs known as bisphosphonates, such as Fosamax (i.e., alendronate), can slow mineral loss, increase bone mass, and reduce the risk of fractures. For patients who cannot take ERT and who have osteoporosis, this is the best treatment available. In some severe cases, physicians prescribe calcitonin, which can slow down the loss of bone minerals.

As noted, weight-bearing exercise slows bone mineral loss. Of course, strenuous activity poses a risk of bone injuries, so people with osteoporosis should consult with their health-care professionals before undertaking such an exercise program.

Analgesics, such as aspirin (*see* page 27), can help relieve pain caused by osteoporosis. Because the greatest danger from this disease involves falls or fractures, treatment for osteoporosis often includes taking measures to prevent injury. Strategies include improving lighting and floor surfaces in the home, adding handrails in the bathroom, and using canes or walkers.

When to seek help.

Seek emergency help if:

- You have a fall or an accident that may have caused a bone fracture.

Call your nurse information service or doctor if:

- You have risk factors for osteoporosis, especially if you are a postmenopausal woman.

PEPTIC ULCER/GASTRITIS

What is a peptic ulcer?

A peptic *ulcer* is an open wound or sore that develops in the mucous membranes (i.e., the membranes that line the body's cavities) of the stomach or the duodenum (i.e., the upper portion of the small intestine). Ulcers developing in the stomach are gastric ulcers; those in the duodenum are duodenal ulcers. Ulcers in the *esophagus* are rare and are not referred to as peptic ulcers.

What causes a peptic ulcer?

To break down food into usable elements, the digestive system uses powerful acids; enzymes, such as pepsin; and hormones, such as gastrin. The membranes that line the surface of the gastrointestinal (GI) system (i.e., the stomach and the intestine) secrete mucus to protect tissues against these corrosive agents. However, excess acid, and irritating drugs (e.g., aspirin), or a disease, such as bacterial infection, can damage these membranes. If this happens, the acids and enzymes can eat away at the unprotected tissue, causing an ulcer.

Roughly 4 out of 5 peptic ulcers (especially duodenal ulcers) probably result from infection by the *Helicobacter pylori* bacterium. Other cases may result from *tumors* that trigger excess production of gastrin, which, in turn, causes the stomach to produce too much acid. Some people inherit a weakness which leads to peptic ulcers. Long-term use of cortisone (i.e., steroid) medications, aspirin (*see* page 27), or nonsteroidal anti-inflammatory drugs (NSAIDs) (*see* page 28) can break down the stomach lining and increase the risk. Despite popular belief, stress and spicy foods do not cause ulcers, but after an ulcer forms, these factors, along with alcohol, caffeine, or smoking, may make it worse. Smoking has been shown to delay the healing of ulcers as well.

What are the symptoms of a peptic ulcer?

Not everyone with a peptic ulcer experiences symptoms. If the ulcer is in the stomach, symptoms typically include a dull, aching pain soon after eating; ulcers in the duodenum can produce a gnawing pain that occurs a few hours after the meal and that may actually be relieved by eating or by drinking milk. Sometimes the pain can radiate (i.e., spread) to the chest or the back. The pain may be present for a few weeks, then subside for a while before recurring. Other symptoms may include indigestion, heartburn, nausea, vomiting, and, in some cases, weight loss.

Severe cases can cause internal bleeding, producing stools that appear black or tarry. Some people may vomit bloody material that resembles coffee grounds. Often, signs of bleeding are noticed before there is any pain. Extreme pain may be a sign of a perforated ulcer, an ulcer that completely penetrates through the lining or wall of the stomach or, more often, the duodenum.

Can a peptic ulcer be prevented?

The bacterium involved in a peptic ulcer is present in most humans by age 60. It is unclear how to avoid infection, but the microbe does not cause ulcers in everyone.

Stopping smoking is the most important step for prevention (*see* page 24). You can also lower your risk by avoiding long-term use of aspirin or NSAIDs. People who have had ulcers before should avoid alcohol, smoking, or foods that have caused symptoms in the past. There is no strong evidence that dietary strategies (e.g., eating small meals more often) do much good. The risk of ulcers is higher in men, among smokers, and in people with a family history of the disease.

How is a peptic ulcer treated?

In mild cases, treatment with drugs that reduce stomach acid or that coat the stomach lining can reduce pain. Many of these products are available without a prescription. Antacids also relieve pain, but they must be taken in low doses to heal the ulcer.

Most ulcers heal after 6 to 8 weeks of treatment, but there is a high risk that ulcers will recur within a year. People who have had ulcers should avoid excessive caffeine (e.g., coffee, tea, cola, and chocolate) or alcohol (*see* page 16). Those who smoke should stop, since smoking contributes to ulcer formation and delays healing (*see* page 24).

Physicians often prescribe an acid reliever, an antacid, and a combination of two antibiotics, such as metronidazole and tetracycline, to cure an underlying bacterial infection if present. If pain persists, gastroscopy (i.e., an examination of the interior of the stomach) is often performed to rule out a more serious cause. These may include a tumor or a buildup of scar tissue, which would require surgery or other treatment options. Because of the many effective treatments available today, surgery is not usually necessary.

When to seek help.

Seek emergency help if:

- You pass bloody or black, tarry stools.
- You experience severe abdominal pain.
- You experience signs of shock (e.g., cold, clammy skin, or fainting).
- You vomit bright red blood.

Call your nurse information service or doctor if:

- You have symptoms of an ulcer that last more than 2 weeks despite self-treatment.

PROSTATE PROBLEM

What is the prostate?

The prostate, found only in men, is a gland about the size and shape of a chestnut, lying just below the bladder and in front of the rectum. It surrounds the *urethra*. The prostate secretes a fluid that becomes part of the semen ejaculated during orgasm.

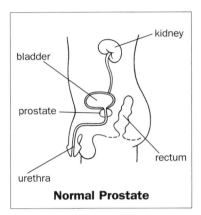

Normal Prostate

What problems can affect the prostate, and what causes them?

Benign prostatic hyperplasia (BPH) means an enlarged prostate. BPH, which is probably triggered by an imbalance in male hormones, is a normal part of aging. It is not *cancerous*.

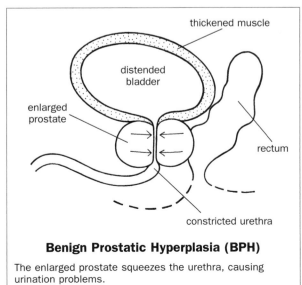

Benign Prostatic Hyperplasia (BPH)

The enlarged prostate squeezes the urethra, causing urination problems.

Prostatitis is an inflammation of the prostate gland, usually caused by bacteria. Prostate cancer is a *tumor* that develops in the prostate. Over time the tumor grows, usually very slowly. If it grows large enough, it may cause symptoms. Cancerous cells can *metastasize,* or spread, to other parts of the body. The exact cause is not known, but male hormones, heredity, and other factors play a part.

What are the symptoms of prostate conditions?

BPH causes problems with urination: weak, hesitant, or interrupted flow; difficulty stopping urine flow; dribbling; or an inability to empty the bladder completely. These symptoms may be worsened by many medications, including cold and allergy pills containing antihistamines and decongestants. Men with BPH typically have to urinate frequently, especially at night, which disrupts sleep. The urge to urinate can be very strong, making it difficult or impossible to postpone urination. Prostatitis can cause blood in the urine or the ejaculate, chills, fever, pain in the lower abdomen or scrotal area, and sometimes painful, difficult urination. Prostate cancer usually causes no symptoms in the early stages. As the tumor grows, urinary problems resembling those seen in BPH may develop. Prostate cancer that has metastasized can cause fatigue, weakness, and pain in the back, ribs, hips, shoulders, or other bones.

Can prostate problems be prevented?

In a word, no. BPH is a fact of life for men; the condition will affect almost all men who live long enough. Prostatitis is an infectious disease, but it is not contagious. It sometimes develops following an infection of the urinary tract or bladder, or following a medical procedure in which a catheter is inserted in the penis. There are no proven strategies for preventing prostate cancer, although some evidence suggests eating a low-fat diet rich in vegetables may provide some protection.

How are prostate problems treated?

If BPH becomes troublesome enough to require treatment, options include prostatectomy and, more commonly, transurethral resection of the prostate (TURP), in which fragments of enlarged prostate tissue are removed using a device inserted through the penis.

Prostatitis caused by bacteria can be treated with antibiotics, such as sulfamethoxazole + trimethoprim or ciprofloxacin, for up to 6 weeks. If the inflammation arises from some other cause, treatment is aimed at relieving symptoms: bed rest, increased fluid intake, and aspirin or other pain relievers (see page 27), and, in some cases where there is obstruction, use of a catheter to help with urination. The treatment of prostate cancer is a complex and controversial subject. In many cases, the tumor will grow so slowly that it will not pose a threat to the man's health or life. For this reason, the option known as "watchful waiting" is worth considering. If a follow-up exam shows that the cancer is growing rapidly, radical prostatectomy is a possibility. Radiation therapy is used to destroy cancerous cells without invasive surgery, but because the prostate remains in the body, it is impossible to know if the treatment is curative. Sometimes a combination of surgery and radiation is recommended. The risks of these methods include incontinence and impotence.

In recent years, a new technique, called brachytherapy, or seed implantation, has been developed; in this approach, radioactive pellets are placed inside the prostate to deliver a more potent dose of radiation directly to the affected cells. Another technique, called cryosurgery, involves the use of a supercold probe to freeze and destroy prostate tissue without the need for surgical removal. Studies are under way to determine whether these methods are as safe and effective as traditional surgery or radiation.

In advanced cases, where the tumor has begun to spread outside the prostate to nearby tissues or other places in the body, hormonal therapy and/or radiation therapy to painful bone metastases is often the only option.

In many cases, doctors will prescribe a combination of these approaches. Choice of treatment depends on many factors: age, general health, cancer stage, and the patient's desires.

When to seek help.

Call your doctor if:

- You have been unable to urinate for more than 12 hours.

Call your nurse information service or doctor if:

- You have trouble urinating or have to get up often during the night to urinate.

- You notice blood in your urine or semen.

SINUSITIS/ALLERGIC RHINITIS

What are sinusitis and allergic rhinitis?

These common conditions involve inflammation of the mucous membranes (i.e, the membranes that line the body's cavities) that line the nose and sinuses (i.e., cavities of the nose and face). Acute sinusitis often arises following a cold or the flu and usually disappears with therapy in 1 to 2 weeks; chronic sinusitis is usually milder, but it lasts longer and recurs throughout the year. Allergic rhinitis (i.e.,"hay fever") is a chronic condition. Some people suffer from symptoms throughout the year, but most experience problems for a few weeks in certain seasons.

What causes sinusitis and allergic rhinitis?

Acute sinusitis often results from a viral infection that weakens the body's defenses and permits a subsequent bacterial infection to take hold. The infection can spread from person to person, or it can arise from an oral infection, such as a tooth abscess. Chronic sinusitis may follow untreated or persistent acute sinusitis, but some cases arise from exposure to airborne irritants, such as dust, chemicals, fumes, or smoke. Cigarette smokers and people with nasal *polyps,* or those born with unusually narrow sinus openings or an abnormality of the nostrils (e.g., deviated septum), are especially susceptible.

Allergic rhinitis develops when the body is sensitive to an allergen, such as pollen, dust, mold, mites, or animal dander (e.g., flakes of skin). Different people are sensitive to different allergens. Because some are allergic to pollen from plants or trees, symptoms may be seasonal, arising when the plants are in bloom (i.e., fall or spring) and receding a few weeks later. Rhinitis may be a response to certain medications, foods, or temperature changes.

What are the symptoms of sinusitis and allergic rhinitis?

In sinusitis, the mucous membranes become inflamed. Swelling blocks the drainage of mucus from the sinuses. Pressure builds up and causes headaches or pain and swelling near the affected sinus: above or behind the eyes, on the bridge of the nose between the eyes, in the cheeks, or in the upper jaw or teeth. The pain may be worse in the morning or when you bend your head down or forward. Sometimes your eyes become watery and the eyelids swell. Typically, you'll have a thick, yellow-green nasal discharge. Blocked nasal passages will force you to breathe through your mouth. You may have fever and chills; sometimes you will lose your sense of smell and taste, and your voice will sound "nasal."

Symptoms of allergic rhinitis resemble those of the common cold: sneezing (sometimes violent and often frequent); nasal congestion and itching; itchy, red, watery eyes; cough or perhaps wheezing; headache; and a persistent tickle in the mouth or throat. You will have a lot of nasal discharge, usually clear and watery. Despite its nickname "hay fever," allergic rhinitis is not usually caused by hay and does not involve fever.

Can sinusitis and allergic rhinitis be prevented?

To reduce the risk of sinusitis, avoid exposure to people with colds. Wash your hands frequently, and avoid touching your nose and eyes. If you get a cold, use a humidifier (or put a saucepan full of water on your radiator) to moisten the air. Drink plenty of liquids, and sleep with your head elevated to promote drainage. Blow your nose gently. Practice good dental hygiene. To minimize outbreaks of allergic rhinitis, use air conditioners or air-purification systems to moisten air and remove allergens. Change the filters on these devices and on furnaces regularly. Stay indoors during peak allergy seasons or on days with high pollen counts. You may need to wear a mask over your nose and mouth. Avoid chores such as dusting, gardening, or mowing the lawn. If you are allergic to your pet, keep the animal clean and groomed and do not allow it in your bedroom. Wash your hair at night and change pillow cases frequently.

How are sinusitis and allergic rhinitis treated?

Most cases of sinusitis can be treated with over-the-counter products. Oral or nasal decongestants and antihistamines (used with caution and as directed by your physician) can reduce swelling and promote drainage. Inhaling steam or using a saline spray can moisten and soothe nasal passages. Analgesics (i.e., pain relievers), ice packs, or heating pads can relieve sinus pain and headache. Your doctor may prescribe antibiotics to eliminate the infection or steroid nasal sprays to reduce inflammation and histamine response. In severe cases, endoscopy (i.e., a procedure used to examine the interior of a body cavity) can clear nasal blockage and surgery can repair sinuses;

long-term (i.e., up to 6 weeks) antibiotics may be needed to get rid of infection.

Allergies can't be cured, but often they tend to get better over time. Antihistamines, short-term use of decongestants, eyedrops, and inhaled or oral corticosteroids can relieve symptoms. Desensitization therapy involves a series of shots to reduce the body's response to allergens. Ask your doctor if this will work for you. Reducing the body's exposure to known allergens is still the best option.

When to seek help.

Seek emergency help if:

- Your eyes appear to bulge or you can't move your eye muscles.

- You experience nausea, vomiting, severe head pain, and high fever.

Call your nurse information service or doctor if:

- Your symptoms lasts for more than 3 days of self-treatment.

- You notice bloody nasal discharge.

STROKE

What is a stroke?

A stroke is brain damage resulting from either an obstruction of the carotid *artery* (located in the neck) or an artery in the head, or a bleed into the brain that destroys nearby delicate brain cells and nerves. Because brain cells cannot regenerate, the damage is often serious and may be permanent. About one third of strokes are fatal. Another term for stroke is cerebrovascular accident. A transient ischemic attack (TIA)—sometimes called a "mini-stroke"—is a temporary arterial blockage that may cause some symptoms but that does not result in brain damage and permanent loss of function.

What causes a stroke?

About 80% of strokes result from blocked arteries. One type of blockage is cerebral thrombosis, in which clots form in the artery and impede the passage of blood. Some strokes arise from cerebral embolism; an embolus—a fragment of material, such as plaque, tissue, or a blood clot—breaks off from elsewhere in the body (e.g., a heart valve, the aorta, or the carotid artery) and travels into an artery in the brain, where it becomes lodged. Other strokes result when an *aneurysm* in an artery wall suddenly ruptures or begins to leak. This type of stroke, known as a cerebral hemorrhage, accounts for about 20% of cases. Bleeding continues until either the pressure stops it or a clot forms and prevents blood from escaping.

Leading risk factors for stroke include high blood pressure (*see* page 244) and atherosclerosis (i.e., narrowed or clogged arteries) (*see* page 236). Age is a major factor; most strokes occur in people over 65. Men are at somewhat higher risk than women. Emboli (plural of embolus) often develop due to

other cardiac illnesses, such as arrhythmias, diseases of the heart valves, myocardial infarction (i.e., heart attack) (*see* page 236), or *cardiomyopathy*. Drugs, such as cocaine or amphetamines, speed up the heart rate and raise blood pressure, increasing the risk. Other risk factors include a history of TIAs; a family history of stroke or heart disease (*see* page 236) and anything that can predispose to *arteriosclerosis*, such as smoking; obesity (*see* page 248); a high-fat, high-cholesterol diet; a sedentary lifestyle; and diabetes (*see* page 240). Oral contraceptives increase the risk of stroke, especially in women over 40 and in cigarette smokers, by making their blood more likely to clot.

What are the warning signs of a stroke?

Strokes occur suddenly and without warning. There may be a severe headache (in the case of a bleed) or loss of consciousness (if a large stroke). Subsequent symptoms depend on the extent and location of damage in the brain. Typical consequences of stroke include:

- Loss of feeling
- Loss of movement
- Tingling sensations in the arms and legs
- Loss of speech or difficulty speaking
- Difficulty swallowing
- Nausea and vomiting
- Vision loss, or vision difficulties (blurred or double vision)
- Mental confusion
- Loss of memory
- Dizziness

Sometimes physical symptoms affect only the right or left side of the body. Symptoms of a TIA include weakness, numbness or tingling, vision problems, speech difficulty, dizziness, and hearing loss.

Can a stroke be prevented?

The best way to prevent stroke is to maintain the healthiest possible lifestyle. Don't smoke (*see* page 24); exercise (*see* page 20); eat a balanced diet low in saturated fats and cholesterol (*see* page 17); keep alcohol consumption to 2 drinks or less per day (*see* page 16). If you are overweight, consider weight-loss strategies (*see* page 25). Ask your physician during your next visit whether you should take aspirin, which is a blood thinner (*see* page 27), regularly as a preventive measure. If you have high blood pressure, follow your doctor's treatment plan. People at risk for stroke, such as those with heart arrhythmias, may benefit from use of medications that prevent blood clots, such as warfarin or ticlopidine. Sometimes a surgical procedure called *carotid endarterectomy* is recommended as a way to clear plaque from the carotid arteries.

How is a stroke treated?

Strokes are medical emergencies. To minimize damage, a stroke victim requires immediate evaluation and hospitalization. If the patient is seen within 6 hours of the stroke and if there is no bleeding risk, strokes resulting from clots may be treated with fast-acting clot-dissolving drugs such as streptokinase, or with anticoagulants such as heparin or warfarin. If an *aneurysm* is involved, emergency treatment is aimed at lowering blood pressure.

After the stroke, steps taken to prevent recurrence include use of blood thinners or anticoagulants to minimize risk of clotting and antihypertensive medications to lower blood pressure. Carotid endarterectomy may be suggested to prevent future strokes.

Other treatments depend on the type and extent of damage caused by the stroke. Many stroke victims need special therapy or assistance to learn how to walk or talk again. Even though brain cells may have been permanently destroyed, it is often possible to "train" other cells to handle certain functions, such as speech or muscle movement. In 1 out of 3 cases, the patient may recover to a greater or lesser extent from damage such as paralysis or loss of speech. In severe cases, around-the-clock, in-home care or a nursing home may be needed.

When to seek help.

Seek emergency help if:

- A person suddenly passes out and does not regain consciousness; has a sudden, persistent loss of strength or speech; or experiences a sudden severe, persistent headache.

Call your nurse information service or doctor if:

- You experience weakness or numbness on one side of the body.

- You fall and don't remember why.

- You suddenly lose vision in one or both eyes.

GLOSSARY

Addison's disease: A disease in which the adrenal glands fail to produce enough steroid hormones; it may result from a problem with the immune system, or from an infection or *tumor*.

allergy: A reaction to a substance which can result in a rash, bronchial congestion, or sneezing due to the release of a chemical called histamine.

amyotrophic lateral sclerosis: A degenerative disease of the motor neurons in the brain and spinal cord that control voluntary muscles.

anaphylaxis: A serious, potentially fatal *allergic* reaction.

aneurysm: A weak spot in an *artery* wall that usually results in a balloon-like swelling.

angina pectoris: A condition in which the heart muscle is deprived of oxygen, causing pain that spreads down the inner left arm; also referred to as angina.

ankylosing spondylitis: An inflammatory disease that primarily affects the spine and causes fusion of joints.

anticoagulant therapy: The administration of drugs to prevent blood clots.

aplastic anemia: A disorder caused by a drop in the production of all types of blood cells in bone marrow.

appendicitis: An inflammation of the appendix.

arrhythmia: An irregular heartbeat.

arteriosclerosis: A disease in which *arteries* lose elasticity, harden, and narrow, resulting in coronary heart disease.

artery: A large blood vessel that carries blood away from the heart to tissue.

aseptic necrosis: A condition in which body tissue stops functioning properly due to an interruption in blood supply (sometimes occurring after an injury).

Bell's palsy: A paralysis of the nerve that goes to the muscles of the face, usually on one side only.

blood clotting disorder: A condition in which the body either cannot halt the flow of blood from a wound by clotting or the blood within the vessels clots too much.

botulism: A type of food poisoning caused by food that has not been properly canned or preserved; produces paralysis and loss of normal sensation.

bronchitis: An inflammation of the bronchial tubes.

brucellosis: A bacterial infection affecting people and animals.

bulimia: An eating disorder characterized by episodes of binge eating, followed by self-induced vomiting.

bullous myringitis: A bacterial infection that causes the formation of small water blisters on the eardrum.

bunion: A thickening of the skin at the base of the big toe caused by poorly fitted shoes.

bunionette: A swelling of the joint at the base of the little toe caused by poorly fitted shoes.

bursitis: An inflammation of bursae, fluid-filled sacs found near joints that reduce friction between tendons and bones; usually affects the shoulder or elbow.

cancer: An uncontrolled growth of malignant (abnormal) cells.

***Candida*:** A yeast infection-causing bacteria; *Candida albicans* is the most common cause.

cardiomyopathy: Any disease affecting the structure and function of the heart.

carotid endarterectomy: A surgical procedure for removing *plaque* blocking the major artery to the brain.

chemotherapy: Any use of chemicals for treatment of disease; most commonly refers to *cancer* treatment.

chlamydia: An infection characterized by painful urination and vaginal or *urethral* discharge.

cholecystitis: An inflammation of the gallbladder that may be caused by gallstones.

chronic cystitis: An inflammation of the urinary bladder.

chronic fatigue syndrome: Severe, chronic, unexplained fatigue.

circulatory problem: An impairment of the body's ability to provide tissue with enough oxygen-rich blood.

cognitive functioning: The ability to make judgments and be aware.

colic: An attack of abdominal pain due to a painful *spasm* or obstruction in one of the hollow, tube-like organs such as the intestine.

collapsed lung: A condition in which air gets into the space around a deflated lung.

concussion: An injury to the head that usually causes a loss of consciousness and is followed by headaches.

cornea: The transparent tissue on the outer wall of the eye through which the iris and pupil can be seen (*see* figure on page 86).

cranial arteritis: An inflammation of the blood vessels in the head.

Crohn's disease: A swelling and inflammation of any part of the intestine, usually at the ileum (the end of the small intestine).

croup: An infection that causes the swelling and narrowing of the large air passages (especially the trachea and larynx); most common in children between the ages of 3 months and 3 years.

cyst: A bag-like growth that can occur anywhere in the body, but is especially common in or under the skin, that contains fluids or semisolid material.

dehydration: A loss of too much water from body tissue.

delayed ejaculation: The failure to ejaculate after having an erection for some length of time; may be caused by anxiety and certain medications.

delusion: A firmly held, irrational belief, not based on reality.

deviated septum: A crooked wall between the nostrils, which narrows the air passage, making breathing difficult.

diabetes acidosis: High acid and ketone levels in the body fluids due to untreated or uncontrolled diabetes; also referred to as diabetic ketoacidosis.

diabetes insipidus: A disorder that results in a loss of the kidney's ability to concentrate urine.

diaphragm: A muscular partition separating the abdomen from the upper part of the chest containing the heart and lungs.

digestive problem: A problem such as heartburn, diarrhea, or indigestion that occurs after eating food.

diphtheria: A serious infection caused by a bacterium, which produces a thick gray membrane on the back of the throat and whose toxin causes inflammation of the heart and nervous system.

dislocation: A result of moving a body part to an unusual position (usually a bone from a joint).

diverticulitis: An inflammation of an abnormal pocket or sac extending from a hollow organ such as the bladder or intestine.

dry mouth: A decrease in the amount of saliva that may result from the use of certain drugs, radiation treatment, or aging.

encephalitis: An inflammation of the brain.

endometrial hyperplasia: A condition in which the lining of the uterus grows too thick, causing abnormal bleeding between menstrual periods and heavy or prolonged menstrual periods.

endometriosis: A condition in which some of the tissue that normally lines the uterus grows in another place, such as the ovary or pelvic wall.

epiglottis: A thin structure located behind the root of the tongue that stops food from being inhaled into the lungs.

epiglottitis: An inflammation of the *epiglottis*.

epilepsy: A disorder of the brain that produces convulsive seizures (fits), lost or altered consciousness, or a variety of neurologic symptoms.

esophageal stricture: A narrowing, or contraction, of the *esophagus*.

esophagus: A tube through which food passes from the mouth to the stomach.

estrogen replacement therapy (ERT): A treatment used to regulate levels of female hormone in women after menopause.

eustachian tube dysfunction: A condition that usually causes a feeling of pressure in the ear and which may rupture the eardrum by stopping the eustachian tube from maintaining the same pressure in the middle and outer ear.

exophthalmos: A condition in which one or both eyeballs stick out abnormally.

flat feet: A condition in which the arches of the feet have flattened out.

flatus: The passage of gas from the rectum.

fracture: A break in a bone.

frostbite: Tissue damage resulting from extreme cold.

gallstones: Stone-like masses, usually consisting of cholesterol, bile pigments, and calcium salts, in the bile duct or gallbladder.

gastritis: An inflammation of the lining of the stomach that may be caused by certain drugs, infections, or excess acid.

giardia: A one-celled organism that causes giardiasis, an infection of the small and/or large intestine.

glossitis: An inflammation of the tongue.

goiter: A swelling in the front part of the neck caused by enlargement of the thyroid gland.

gonorrhea: A bacterial infection characterized by painful urination and yellowish pus-like discharge from the vagina or penis; it is usually sexually transmitted.

gravel: Small concentrations of mineralized salts; smaller than "stones" of the kidney or bladder.

hallucination: The perception of objects that are not really there.

head cold: A contagious, minor illness resulting from a viral infection.

heart block: An abnormal electrical conduction to heart tissue, which may result in a slowed heartbeat.

heart palpitation: A sudden change in the rhythm of the heartbeat.

heat exhaustion: An illness due to heat exposure or inability to adjust to heat.

Helicobacter pylori: A bacterium that causes *ulcers* and *gastritis*.

hemolytic anemia: The destruction of red blood cells; occurs with some infections, inherited disorders, and drug reactions.

hepatitis: A disease in which the liver becomes inflamed.

Hodgkin's lymphoma: A *tumor* of the lymph system, generally beginning with a painless enlargement of lymph glands in the neck.

hormonal disorder: An abnormal level of chemicals produced from a gland, such as the thyroid, pancreas, or reproductive organs.

hot flash: A sudden sensation of warmth and flushing.

hydrocephalus: An abnormal accumulation of fluid in and around the brain.

hypercalcemia: An abnormally high concentration of calcium in the blood.

hypoglycemia: A condition in which glucose (sugar) levels in the blood are low enough to cause symptoms.

hypothermia: A lower than normal body temperature, usually caused by prolonged exposure to cold, which can be a serious or life-threatening condition.

impacted tooth: A tooth poorly positioned within the jaw so that it can't grow through the gum normally.

incontinence: An inability to control urination and/or bowel movements.

infectious arthritis: Arthritis usually due to bacteria that are causing an infection in the joints or elsewhere in the body.

influenza: An infectious respiratory disease caused by a virus.

intestinal obstruction: A blockage of the intestine that prevents passage of the bowel's contents, due to a protrusion, scar tissue, impacted feces, or *tumor.*

intestinal parasite: An organism that invades the intestines, such as a tapeworm, hookworm, or microscopic organism.

iritis: An inflammation of the iris.

juvenile rheumatoid arthritis: A form of rheumatoid arthritis affecting children under age 16.

kidney failure: A condition in which the kidneys stop eliminating wastes due to damage caused by toxic agents, immune reactions, or certain infections or other diseases (especially diabetes).

leukemia: An uncontrolled, malignant (abnormal) growth of white blood cells in bone marrow.

lupus erythematosus: A chronic inflammatory disease that affects blood vessels, kidneys, joints, skin, and the nervous system.

lymphoma: A malignant (abnormal) growth of lymphoid tissue.

macular degeneration: A progressive breakdown of the vascular membrane and retinal cells that are responsible for vision.

malnutrition: A nutritional disorder resulting from a history of unbalanced, insufficient meals, or from poor absorption of foods by the gut.

mastoiditis: An inflammation of the round bone behind the ear.

measles: A highly contagious viral infection that affects the respiratory tract.

metabolism: The sum of all the physical and chemical processes that create and maintain a living organism.

metastasis: The spread of cancerous cells to other sites.

multiple sclerosis: A disease of the central nervous system, caused by loss of myelin (a protective covering) around nerve fibers of the brain and spinal cord, that affects nerve function.

myocarditis: An inflammation of the heart muscle.

narcolepsy: A condition characterized by sudden, uncontrollable, brief episodes of sleep.

neuralgia: A sudden, shooting, usually intense pain along a nerve.

neuropathy: An inflammation or degeneration of nerves.

nodule: A small, rounded, solid mass of tissue.

optic neuritis: An inflammation, deterioration, or loss of myelin (a protective covering) around the optic nerve, which affects vision.

oral lichen planus: Small, pale pimples or shiny, raised patches appearing on the sides of the tongue or inside the cheeks.

osteomyelitis: A painful inflammation of bone marrow or bone caused by infection due to bacteria.

otitis media: An inflammation of the middle ear caused by infection; common in children.

otosclerosis: A disorder caused by an abnormal growth of spongy bone at the entrance to the inner ear, resulting in gradual hearing loss.

parasitic infection: An infection or disease caused by organisms that invade the body and live either on or in it.

Parkinson's disease: A degenerative disorder of a part of the brain, characterized by trembling and muscle rigidity.

partial gastrectomy: A method of treating peptic *ulcer* or *cancer* by removing the part of the stomach that produces digestive acid.

perforated eardrum: A puncture of the membrane leading from the ear canal to the middle ear.

periodontitis: An inflammation of the gums which, if left untreated, can destroy tissue and may ultimately lead to the loss of teeth.

peritonitis: An inflammation of the lining of the abdominal cavity.

pertussis: An infectious, bacterial disease that usually affects children and causes a convulsive cough; also referred to as "whooping cough."

Peyronie's disease: A curvature of the penis that usually affects men between the ages of 40 and 60.

plantar fasciitis: A pain in the sole of the foot, often caused by overuse, which results in inflammation; pain is usually worse in the morning and diminishes as the foot stretches out.

plaque: An elevated, abnormal area caused by disease or injury.

pleurisy: An inflammation of the membrane that covers the lungs and chest cavity.

pneumonia: An infection and inflammation of the lungs.

pneumothorax: A condition in which air in the chest cavity causes lung collapse.

polymyalgia rheumatica: A condition seen in adults over age 50 and characterized by pain and stiffness, especially of the shoulder and hips.

polyp: A *tumor* that is usually benign.

porphyria: An inherited disorder that affects enzymes (proteins) that are involved in the formation of heme (the oxygen-carrying protein in red blood cells).

proctitis: An inflammation of the rectum.

prolapsed disk: A condition in which the cushion-like material between the vertebrae (bones of the spine) moves out of place and may press on nerves; also referred to as a "slipped disk."

presbycusis: Age-related hearing loss.

pseudogout: A condition in which calcium deposits form within the joints, especially the knees.

pulmonary embolus: A blood clot, air bubble, or other foreign deposit in the lungs.

pustule: A small, blister-like elevation of the skin that contains white blood cells or pus.

quinine: A crystalline alkaloid that has medicinal properties; it is used to treat malaria and nightime muscle cramps, and is found in antipyretics (fever reducers).

radiotherapy: The treatment of disease using electromagnetic radiation.

refraction error: A condition in which the reflected light from objects is not focused properly through the eye, causing nearsightedness or farsightedness.

retinal detachment: A separation of the retina (cell layer on the back of the eye) from the blood vessels underneath it.

retinal vessel occlusion: A condition in which a vein or *artery* attached to the retina (cell layer on the back of the eye) becomes blocked.

rotator cuff tear: An injury to the tendons associated with the shoulder joint.

salivary gland disorder: A salivary gland malfunction, due to aging, infection, or the use of certain drugs, that may result in excessive or decreased thirst.

sciatica: A pain in the lower back and hips that radiates down the back of the thighs and into the legs, usually caused by a herniated disk pushing on the sciatic nerve.

scoliosis: A curving of the spine.

sensorineural loss: A loss of hearing due to a defect in the inner ear; patients with this type of hearing loss may be helped with a hearing aid.

shingles: An infection caused by the same virus that causes chicken pox; also referred to as herpes zoster.

sickle cell anemia: A hereditary condition that mainly affects people of African descent, in which abnormal, crescent-shaped red blood cells block blood flow to tissue.

spasm: An involuntary movement resulting from muscle contractions.

spleen: An oval, spongy organ in the upper left part of the abdomen, tucked under the ribs, next to the *diaphragm*. It is important as an aid in fighting many types of infections.

spondylosis: A condition in which the spine slowly loses flexibility and becomes stiff.

sputum: The mucus expelled by clearing the throat or coughing.

stomach-acid reflux: A backward flow of acid from the stomach into the *esophagus*, which may cause heartburn or other illnesses.

strabismus: An impairment of eye muscles or nerves that results in misalignment of the eyes; sometimes referred to as "crossed eyes" or "lazy eye."

stye: An inflammatory, bacterial infection of the sebaceous glands of the eyelids.

synovium: A membrane at the joint between two bones; it produces synovial fluid, which lubricates the moving part of a joint.

tendon: The connective tissue that attaches muscles to bones and other parts.

tetanus: An infectious disease caused by bacteria that usually enter the body through a puncture wound.

thyroiditis: An inflammation of the thyroid gland.

tuberculosis (TB): An infection that affects the lungs.

tumor: An abnormal growth of tissue.

ulcer: An open sore or scarring on the surface of tissue that may be shallow or deep.

ulcerative colitis: A chronic disease characterized by diarrhea, inflammation, and *ulcers* of the colon and rectum.

ultraviolet: That part of the spectrum of sunlight that stimulates production of vitamin D, kills certain bacteria, and causes sunburn and skin damage which can lead to skin *cancer*.

urethra: The tube that allows the passage of urine from the bladder to the body's exterior.

uterine fibroid: A *tumor* attached to the uterine wall that may cause heavy or prolonged menstrual periods and lower abdominal pain, but is often asymptomatic (without symptoms).

uveitis: An inflammation of the iris.

vaginitis: An inflammation of the vaginal tissue.

varicose veins: Enlarged veins close to the skin, most often in the lower legs; they may cause pain in the feet and ankles and are made worse by pregnancy, obesity, and standing for long periods of time.

vertebra: One of the disk-shaped bones of the spine.

Wegener's granulomatosis: A disease in which *nodular* inflammatory lesions (abnormal areas) appear in the upper respiratory tract.

Wilson's disease: A rare, inherited condition in which cirrhosis (scarring) of the liver occurs and the brain's tissues degenerate.

INDEX